Fly With Me

A True Story of Healing from Multiple Sclerosis

Helen Phillips

authorHOUSE®

AuthorHouse™ UK Ltd.
500 Avebury Boulevard
Central Milton Keynes, MK9 2BE
www.authorhouse.co.uk
Phone: 08001974150

First published by AuthorHouse 9/4/2009

ISBN: 978-1-4490-0111-7 (sc)

This book is printed on acid-free paper.

Contents

The Author

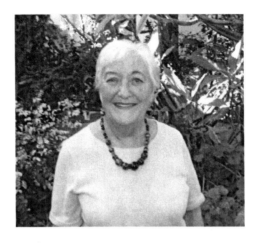

Helen Phillips was diagnosed with Multiple Sclerosis when she was 27 years old and a mother of 3 young children. This is her true story of suffering with MS, the long lessons for healing and trials in war, widowhood, remarriage, divorce and financial struggle.

Helen was born in South Africa, and educated in Rhodesia (now Zimbabwe). She went to university in Cape Town, South Africa, but married before she completed her degree. She and her husband moved back to Rhodesia in 1967 where she became ill and was diagnosed with Multiple Sclerosis. She and her family went through the Rhodesian civil war, her husband died in Harare in 1977 and she moved back to Cape Town with her children.

She is now involved in community work with the poor in Muizenberg, Cape Town and writes and paints in her spare time. She also does relief work at the Christian

Radio Station CCFm and with her husband distributes food for the poor on behalf of her church.

Dedication

I wish to dedicate this book to

My husband Bill,

My children

Kenneth, Douglas, Joy and Ramsay and their respective
spouses

And my grandchildren

Kara, Daniel, Nicola, Daniel George, James and Clair

Psalm 9; 13b-14

Rescue me from death, Lord,
That I may stand before the people of Zion
And tell them all the things for which I praise you.
I will rejoice because you saved me.

The Psalms for Modern Man
Today's English Version

Preface

By Pastor John Thomas

King of Kings Baptist Church, Fish Hoek, South Africa

Helen's painful testimony is written in a gripping style. You don't want to put this down once you start. As you read you feel as if you want to go to the last chapter to see whether it all ends well. For anyone who is sick and trusting God for a miraculous healing this is a must read. She describes the roller coaster ride of faith and doubt as well as the hope and scepticism of well meaning Christians. Her testimony of the journey of her healing is also a good theological treatise on the subject of healing. Her honesty is fantastic as she shares her spiritual growth through many different experiences. Her life testimony of coping with family traumas, war, divorce, dealing with anger and depression, forgiveness, remarriage and finding work will encourage you to put your faith in a great God who is able and meets every need, some of them in surprising ways. You are not going to agree with everything in this book,

but it is an extremely honest story of the ups and downs
of life which all Christians face.

Pastor John Thomas
B.A.hons (Psych) Licentiate Theology.
Past President Baptist Union
Chairman Living Hope

Pastor Jeff Kidwell
The Bay Community Church
Muizenberg

This is not a book for sceptics. This is a book for those who want to believe that the God that we serve is able to do abundantly more than we could ever ask or imagine. And He did just that through the persevering faith of a woman who dared to believe Him.

Helen tells it like it is, that's the Helen I know, and as you read this story, you will be challenged in your faith, but you will be blessed by her honesty, her determination, and her growing understanding of the great God of love and miracles that we serve.

Pastor Jeff Kidwell
The Bay Community Church

Foreward

This is a true story of the amazing things God has done in my life. I could have gone on longer but I did not want to detract from the main reason for writing it. God loves us, protects us and He Heals. He heals all situations but it is not always an instantaneous healing and He works in us, drawing us closer into Himself.

None of the people in this book are fictitious but I have left out some surnames of people who wish to remain anonymous. Tony, the Anglican Minister in Gatooma said so many miracles of healings happened after I left, that people were looking to him and not to God, and he did not want that happening again.

I wish to thank my husband, Bill, for the time he put into editing this book. Without his continuous support, encouragement and honest comment I don't think it would have been done. My friend, Ann Swanepoel has also given me invaluable help with encouragement, editing, and suggestions.

I also wish to thank those who have sponsored the publication for this book; Percy Macaskill, Ann Swanepoel, June Gray, Bea Mannering and members of the Bay Community Church.

Thanks go also to Pastor John Thomas who encouraged me to persevere and complete the revision of this book.

Our Pastor Jeff Kidwell and his wife Viv have been a constant support and I wish to thank them for their spiritual guidance, friendship and prayers.

My main thanks go to God. He is so good and His mercy endures forever.

HelenPhillips
Muizenberg, Cape Town, South Africa 2009

Chapter 1.

Help! I can't walk

Gatooma, (now Gadoma) was a quaint little town in Rhodesia (now Zimbabwe). My husband, Malcolm, and I and our two lovely little boys had moved there in 1967.

The single hotel had a sign in reception "All rooms facing the sea". There was no sea for 2000 miles; the surrounding countryside was dry and dusty bushveld with thorn trees, Mopani and Msasa trees and tall dry grass. The people of Gatooma loved that sign. We were proud of our funny little town.

We had come to Zimbabwe to buy a farm as land was too expensive for us in our homeland, South Africa. Malcolm had not found just what he wanted, so had taken a job as an agricultural representative and we settled in Gatooma while he continued to look around. A beautiful daughter was added to our family in 1968 and I was a happy young lady looking after family, home and garden while Malcolm drove around the countryside selling fertilizer and veterinary products to the local farmers.

I had other interests as well, played tennis three times a week and was runner up in the club championships. I learned to play bridge and while we were sorting out clubs and spades, our children were playing with buckets and spades under the watchful eyes of their nannies. It was a great social time for all of us, moms, children and nannies.

Malcolm opened an agency to market his products and I added a home and garden section and worked there in the mornings. I had no qualifications as I had married after first year university but I had all the enthusiasm and drive to make up for my lack of expertise and soon learned how to run the shop.

I was one of the two organists at the Anglican church and was on the church council. I did the flowers in the church and anything else that needed to be done. It was good to be busy and useful and I was happy.

I was a true Christian, believed in my heart and loved my Lord, but I had never heard the term 'Born Again'. My Bible knowledge was limited but I spent hours practising my hymns, singing along and worshipping God at the same time.

I had grown up as an only child and my mother had taught me about her Jesus and, as a little girl, I would talk to Him while playing alone in the garden, making stick dolls and dressing them with flowers and leaves. I spent many solitary hours pouring over picture books of the life of Jesus and He was very real to me. I knew that He was there with me all the time and I could talk to Him as my companion. Jesus was my friend.

My confirmation and first communion meant a tremendous amount to me and I know now that I was born again at that time. Mine was a simple childlike faith which was part of me and my life. I was truly blessed.

The first time I felt the touch of Jesus, and it was a literal touch, was when I was thirteen. My parents had moved to Bulawayo, Zimbabwe, and had to go out to a Rotary function one night. I was left securely locked in our home at the Hillside Dams but I was afraid of the dark.

I had had a nasty experience in Springs, South Africa, when I was six and woke one night to find a burglar at my bedroom window hooking the blankets off my bed. I was terrified and had never got over the fear of that moment. This time, however, my parents could not take me with them and surely now at thirteen I was old enough to stay on my own. We all thought so. I would be brave.

I was trying to get to sleep after saying my prayers when the front door bell rang. I was terrified. I went stiff and cold with fear and could not move.

The bell rang twice more and I knew I must get up and answer. I was shaking and moved stiff legged but managed to get out of bed. The door bell rang again and I stumbled to the locked passage door but could not even put out my hand to open it. I stood there frozen with fear.

At last I remembered my God.
"Jesus, please help me." I whispered.
Immediately I felt a soft touch on my shoulder and a great peace came over me. I knew that Jesus was with me, had His hand on my shoulder and that I would be safe. I was not alone.

The anti climax of the story was that there was a policeman at the door. He was lost and was just asking for directions.
I could feel God smiling at me and saying, "See, I would not let anything bad happen to you."
If there were any burglars around, they would have made off with the appearance of a policeman. Maybe that was why God sent him around.

Yes, I knew that God was real but in the hectic happy life in Gatooma, I didn't spend the time with Him that I should have. I was too busy.

Then one morning I woke up and I could not walk.

It was very early, the dawn was just breaking and a few sleepy birds were chirping. My daughter, Joy, eighteen months old then, was calling from her cot in the next room, calling to be picked up for her morning cuddle. I lay still hoping she would go back to sleep but she soon started crying and I was forced to move. I didn't want her waking the whole household at that early hour.

I jumped out of bed in my normal energetic way and landed on the floor. I had no sensation of falling. It was as if the floor came up to meet me.

This was weird, I thought. I must be still half asleep. I pulled myself back onto the bed and tried again. Again I fell down. I tried again and once again I fell down.

Joy was really crying now and I knew I must do something. When baby cries, mother must go.

I crawled to the wall and pulled myself up and walking crablike with my hands on the wall, made my way to the next room. I hung onto the door and supporting myself along the wall, shuffled to her cot and with one arm lifted her down and she toddled off to my bed.

Now I had to get back. I made my way slowly the way I had come but when I saw my bed across the room, I thought what nonsense this was and I let go the wall to walk. Down I went again and landed on the floor.

Then I realized that there was something wrong, awfully wrong. I could not walk.

Malcolm called the doctor and he said he could find nothing wrong. He said I was probably overdoing it and all I needed was rest but he took blood tests to make sure. My friends all came to tea and with much hilarity we decided I was shamming and this was just an excuse to be waited on hand and foot.

Next day the doctor came again with the results of the blood tests. My uric acid was high and so I must have some sort of gout.

Now my friends really roared with laughter. We all did. Here I was 27years old, slim as a whistle, fit as a fiddle and a non drinker with gout which, we thought, was only an old fat, drinking man's problem. It was the joke of the town. In a small town of 3000 people news travels fast and I was labelled amongst my friends and acquaintances, as 'Helen with gout'.

Gradually I got better and could walk haltingly but I never went back to tennis and my fingers would not work to play the piano or organ. The church had been praying for me and even when I was well enough to go to church, they still prayed for me. It was quite embarrassing and I told Tony, our minister, that he could stop now as I was back in the congregation.

He said they would go on praying for me until I was one hundred percent fit again. I thought they were just praying to get their organist back as Pat, the other organist, needed a break. Now I thank God for the faithful prayers of the church.

Other peculiar things started happening to my body. I got pins and needles in patches on my legs and when they went away, I felt as if I had ants crawling all over me, dizzy ants going round and round driving me wild. Then the itches started. All of a sudden I would get an itch on my nose and would have to scratch frantically until it went away and came back on my scalp or my neck. I was scratching as if I had fleas. Then I got cramps between my ribs. What a stupid place to get cramp! You could do nothing but hang on to the knot of muscles until they loosened again.

The second attack came about three months later and this time it was very much worse. I had a horrific pain in my neck (gout?) and I could not move my head to look around at all. Not only could I not stand or walk but I could not use my hands at all. I could not hold a cup, pen, knife or fork; buttons were the worst and I could not dress myself properly. I lost sensation on the right hand side of my body and could not feel anything, not even hot or cold temperatures..

As a family we laughed about it. We all thought it was hilarious when mummy couldn't even feed herself properly. Even Joy could do better than I. I jammed the fork against my cheek and spilled everything. Ouch! I didn't know till then that the tips of a fork are sharp and hurt when you missed your mouth. I now know why we give babies plastic covered spoons! I had to laugh to keep things light-hearted for the children's sake.

Beneath my laughter, however, I was starting to feel afraid. This was no fun. Malcolm had to bath and dress me. Underclothes were a major challenge. Even raising my arms to get a dress on was impossible. Kenneth, my eldest son, had to lift my arms one by one while Malcolm had to slip the dress over them. Only people, who have had experience of dressing others, know the complicated manoeuvres needed! It was most awkward.

My own doctor, who had been on sabbatical in England when I had had the first attack, came to see me. He asked me to put my finger on my nose with my eyes closed. It was like pinning the tail on the donkey blindfolded at a children's party. I felt so foolish but could not do it. I had to try and walk on a line but, of course, I fell over.

The doctor looked grave and said he wanted me to go to St Anne's Hospital in Harare to see a specialist. The children were parcelled out to friends and Malcolm drove me through. Now I was really afraid and Malcolm said very little but he was obviously very worried. The horror, for me, was being so helpless and dependent and not knowing what was wrong. We never spoke of it. It was too much.

St Anne's was a lovely, light airy hospital with smiling nuns who were very kind but I felt so alone, away from my friends and family. I asked for a minister to come and see me but although the nuns said they had phoned, nobody came. I tried to read my bible and pray but I just couldn't get through. My fear was consuming me.

I thought I would go to the chapel and see if that would help me to pray and find God. I refused a wheelchair but pulled myself along the beds and walls of the corridors. I was exhausted by the time I got there and sat down in the little gallery to catch my breath but my soul found no peace.

I had never been into a church like this before and it was foreign and different. The chapel was beautiful with flowers and stained glass windows but when I saw people genuflecting and lighting candles in front of life-size statues, I felt so out of place. There was an unbearable loneliness in my soul and a yearning for a more personal encounter with Him. I remained comfortless and stumbled back to my ward feeling more alone than ever. I could not find my God.

I now know that my fear was separating me from God and He could not get through to me in this panic, but at the time I felt abandoned and I was desperate for Him.

The specialist did innumerable tests, blood tests, ECGs and EEGs, lumbar punctures and myelograms. He pricked me, poked and stroked me with feathers, cotton wool and pins all up my arms and legs and face and I had to tell him what I felt.

"Can you feel this? Is it soft and tickly or smooth? Can you feel this prick? Is my pin sharp or blunt? Does it hurt?"
He tapped my knees and ankles with reflex hammers and tickled me under my feet till I wanted to scream.
The specialist physician called in the neurosurgeon. There was no neurologist in Harare. They wanted to know all about the first attack and the dead feelings on the left hand side of my body, the first time, and the right hand side, the second time. They wanted to know about the pins and

needles, the ants and spiders crawling, the cramps and the itches. It felt as if they wanted to know about every sneeze. They were thorough but it is difficult to describe some things, like the feeling of having thick gloves on my hands. They nodded and looked grave and went off to confer without telling me anything.

I had to try to lift my legs while they held them down. I had to hold their arms and try to pull myself up. Of course my arms and legs would not work properly.

They asked me where in England I was born.

"I was born in South Africa," I replied.

"Are you sure? Are you sure you were not born in England?"

As if I didn't know where I was born.

"How is your eye sight?"

"Fine."

"Can you see out of the sides of your eyes?"

I moved my eyes around. "Yes I can see."

"Are you sure? Can you see when I wiggle my finger like this?"

"Yes, I can."

This was not '20 Questions' but 101 questions. They went on and on repeating themselves.

It was annoying but quite amusing until I started to realize what they were probing for.

Malcolm had a friend, Ray Shaw, who lived in the Eastern Transvaal where we had lived when we were first married. We used to visit him regularly. Ray was 35, in a wheelchair, his peripheral vision had failed first and now he had about

6% of his sight. His bowels and bladder had stopped functioning so he had had to have a colostomy and also used a catheter and bag. Although his speech was slurred and he tired quickly, his lovely nature and personality shone through it all. He had told us all about his illness and how rare it was in people born in South Africa although it was relatively common in England. In South Africa it normally only attacked people born in England.

Ray had Multiple Sclerosis. It was an almost unknown disease at that time. Previously doctors had thought it was some sort of mental condition that drove patients to fake paralysis.

I also had an uncle who had had Multiple Sclerosis. I had seen him battling to walk and still run a farm. He had been diagnosed when he was middle aged and he had died within about 6 years.

My horror and fear increased with every test and question. I did not mind dying as I knew I would be with my Lord Jesus, but I did mind leaving my family and I did not ever want to land up in a wheelchair like Ray. Imagine not being able to read or even hold a book. Imagine never being able to dress or bath myself or go to the toilet. I couldn't and did not want to begin thinking about it.
"Please, Lord, never. I want to be with my children and family but please, Lord, never in that condition." I prayed.

Eventually I plucked up the courage and asked the doctors what was wrong with me.
"I am afraid we cannot tell you," they said.

"Then what are you looking for?" I asked.

They looked at each other. "No, we don't want to tell you that either."

I was desperate and indignant. "This is my body. I have every right to know what is wrong with me."

"We would rather not tell you, yet"

"I am a Christian," I said, "and have God to rely on so I have strength to handle it. Tell me, please. What do you think this is?'

They shook their heads and were about to walk away as my fear grew to panic.

"If I guess, will you tell me yes or no?" I called after them.

They looked at each other and came back beside my bed. "OK, that's fair."

"Have I got Multiple Sclerosis?"

The shocked look on their faces told me all I needed to know. The disease was so rare especially in Zimbabwe at that time, they never dreamt I would guess correctly. When they nodded their heads sadly and said yes, that is what they thought, I was shattered. I thought it would help knowing the truth but I kept on seeing Ray in my mind's eye. I could not get like that. I WOULD NOT get like that.

Malcolm went to pieces when he was told and when he came to fetch me, his eyes were blood shot and drooping and I could see that he had been drinking heavily. This did not make me feel any better. If my husband could not take the news, how could he support me in this illness? I felt angry and more alone than ever.

We did not talk about it or say much at all. We drove back to Gatooma thinking our own tortuous thoughts, wondering what the future held for each of us. I had an incurable disease which would destroy my body and Malcolm had a wife who would be both paralyzed and blind.

Fear and panic churned in both of us.

Chapter 2

Amazing Heat

As we drove into our driveway a couple of hours later a car drew up behind us. It was Tony, the Anglican minister. He was a big man, six foot six inches tall and strong, with fiery auburn hair.

Before I could open my door, he was beside the car with a warm smile.
"Hi there," he said. "I phoned the hospital in Salisbury and they told me what time you had left. How's that for timing?"

He picked me up like a baby and carried me inside, depositing me on the settee in the lounge. Malcolm collapsed into a chair nearby.
Tony did not sit but towered above us.

"I have known all along what was wrong with you," he said quietly. "Multiple Sclerosis is quite common in England and I know quite a few people who have it. I have been praying for you and God has told me that you must kneel down here, on the carpet in the lounge, and I must lay hands on you and He will heal you."

Malcolm and I looked at him in surprise. This was an Anglican and our religion was very private and personal. We did not do things like that back in 1969.

"Yes, this is a first for me too," he said, "but the message is clear and we must do it."

He and Malcolm helped me down to kneel on the floor, leaning against a chair, and he laid his hands on my head and started to pray.

Well, I have never known anything like it nor will I ever again I suppose. The heat was absolutely amazing.

This heat that came from Tony's hands was much hotter than human heat, yet it did not burn. It flooded me from the top of my head, spreading down through my neck, back, body and legs, right down to my feet. I could feel its gentle but strong movement like hot oil, soothing and warming yet vibrant, powerful and alive. I don't know how else to describe it.

It was wonderful. It was the touch of the Holy Spirit of God and His healing power.

I don't know what Tony prayed. I did not even hear as I revelled in the amazing sensation and wondered in awe.

The dreadful pain in my neck went immediately and my fear disappeared completely, to be replaced by an absolute peace; a certainty that this was the touch of God and I had nothing to worry about because He was healing me.

This was the tangible reality of the presence of the loving, almighty God I had been searching for in the chapel in hospital. This was wonderful!

How long we remained in that position, I do not know. I did not want it to end. I was bathed and basking in this amazing healing warmth of God. Tony said later his hands were so hot that they were burning, but he could not move them.

A tremendous joy welled up inside me. I was glowing. I was smiling from ear to ear and the panic that had consumed me had totally gone. I was in a warm bubbling place and so happy.

I have never been the same since.

The truth is that in the natural, my pain had gone, but I still could not walk, dress or feed myself. The paralysis was still there but **I** was changed. Now instead of fear, I had complete faith, joy and peace. I knew absolutely, that God was healing me and I put myself totally in His hands. It did not matter that I couldn't walk or do anything for myself. I was in God's hands and I **would** be well again.

I had such an inner certainty that I thought it merely amusing when Kenneth's school teacher came to visit me and told me her experience of this disease in England. "Don't worry, my dear," she said, "You will only be permanently in a wheel chair when your children are teenagers. It progresses very slowly."

I tried to tell her that I was being healed but she looked at me with such pity that I smiled and chuckled in my heart, feeling sorry for her because she did not know, nor had ever experienced, the wonderful touch of God. When I tried to explain it to her she looked at me blankly. She did not understand at all.

The Baptist minister, who was another friend, came to visit me and pray with me. He was nonplussed by my happiness as he was prepared to give me words of comfort.

My friends on the whole were very sorry for me and embarrassed about the whole thing. After visiting me once or twice, they stopped coming as they did not know what to say. No one believed that I was healed as I was still totally incapacitated. Everyone thought I was deluded and in denial. Here I sat and could do nothing but I believed I was being healed by God. They thought it all very strange.

I was singing and joyful in my heart against all odds. It was not put on. It was not an act to conjure up faith to be healed. This was the faith of God which **He** had given me and it was amazing. God is so wonderful. It was all His doing, not my faith but His. I did nothing but allow Him to work in me.

Even Tony was a bit perplexed by the whole thing. He said to me that euphoria was a symptom of the disease in some people but I laughed at him.

"You think this is euphoria? This is God!! Isn't it amazing and wonderful? I have never been happier in my life. I never knew God could be so wonderful. I am a different person, my whole life is different. Yes, I am touched in the head, touched by God."

Malcolm looked on puzzled and said nothing. The children were so pleased to have mummy singing and happy even if she could still do nothing but sit. They would come and sit with me and I would read and talk to them and tell them Jesus was making me better.

The old chorus says it so well:

> *It's bubbling, it's bubbling,*
> *It's bubbling in my soul,*
> *It's singing and laughing*
> *Since Jesus made me whole.*
> *Folks don't understand it*
> *Nor can I tell them why,*
> *It's bubbling, bubbling, bubbling,*
> *Bubbling, bubbling*
> *Day and night.*

Tony was wonderfully supportive. Looking back, I know he didn't have the same kind of faith that I did. Maybe he felt that my faith was euphoric but he never undermined it and he fed me with every book he could get about God's healing. There was nothing else I could do, as I could not walk or do anything, so I sat on the couch in my bedroom looking out at the beautiful garden and I read and I studied.

I drank in everything like a thirsty sponge.

I rationalized it this way. I had an incurable disease. Doctors did not know what to do and could do nothing for me but God knew everything and could do anything. He had healed when He walked this earth and I would go to Him as my doctor.

I embarked on a full Bible study on healing. What did God say about healing?

What did He say about sickness and where did he put Himself in the fight against disease?

Where did sickness come from? Did God bring sickness if He was almighty and reigned?

I sat with my concordance and several different versions of the bible and lost myself in studying and listening to God.

I did not know my Bible well and it was an exciting journey delving into it now. I discovered in Exodus chapter 15 verse 26 that He says He is our Healer. In the psalms He says that no sickness will come near us and we need not fear as

'He will deliver us from the deadly pestilence' (Psalm 91 ; 3). I found references all over the Bible and combined with the healings that Jesus did on Earth I knew that God was confirming His word and His actions.

Friends brought me books on healing. Some I rejected as not being in line with God's word but others I absorbed and put into practice.

I learned to put myself into God's presence in my mind and imagination, basking in His light and warmth. I wanted to learn more and more about God and what I must do to manifest His healing so others could see it.

One day when I was reading the gospel of John and came to chapter 15, I realized that this is what I had to do. Later God confirmed this for me by giving me a vision and similar modern parable.

John 15 says we are the branches of the vine, the Father is the farmer, Jesus is the vine, so the Holy Spirit is the sap flowing from the roots to the branch. I was the branch and I just had to stay in the stem. I couldn't jump off the vine or I would die and I did not have to struggle to stay in the vine or work hard to be there, I just had to **be.** The sap of the vine would pass into me in the normal natural process and that was the Comforter, the Helper, the Healing Life of God.

God taught me to pray and think in pictures. I saw myself playing tennis again, running and smashing those balls.. I saw myself climbing onto His lap as a little girl, just as He said to his disciples, "Let the little children to come to me." I felt myself snuggling down in warmth and security with His arms around me.

I did not know the necessity of faith at the beginning but the pictures gave me a certainty of things to come, a certainty of my healing. Now I know that the Bible says that faith is the evidence, the realisation and assurance of things hoped for, the conviction of things not seen. (Hebrews 11.1)

He showed me strolling in the garden and planting new plants, picking flowers and arranging them in the house, playing with my children, swimming with them, running around and throwing balls to them. All things that I loved to do. With every picture my spirits soared and I got excited about what I would be doing when I could walk again. I did not know it then, but by these pictures held in my mind, and all prompted by God, He was teaching me faith. I had **His** faith by the tremendous experience of His healing anointing, but He was giving me even more to hang on to. He was teaching me to **see** my healing.

As Jesus said, 'The Holy Spirit will be your teacher.'

I needed this faith as I was tested and tried over and over again by other people's unbelief and God put into my mind all these pictures of me healed, to build my faith.

Soon I was to be tested almost to breaking point.

Chapter 3

Too Happy

My parents in Cape Town were understandably very concerned and worried about me and my father insisted that I fly down to Groote Schuur Hospital to the neurology professor, to get a second opinion. He also found a private neurologist, Dr Thorne, who had just returned from England, where he had made a study of Multiple Sclerosis. Dad did not believe that his beloved only child had this incurable disease.

My mother flew up to Zimbabwe to look after the children and I flew down to Cape Town.

The trip was terrible. I had always refused a wheelchair before. It seemed an admission of defeat so I would get along hanging onto things and people, but you can't do that at a big international airport. I had to have a wheelchair.

For those who have never had to be in a wheelchair let me tell you it is the most demeaning experience. All of a sudden people treat you as if you are not there, or as a child to be noticed occasionally. They talk over your head and talk about you in the third person, he, she or it. I felt like an 'it' after a little while. Everybody looked at me with pity, or embarrassment and I felt completely depersonalized. Don't ever give me a wheelchair again. I am now very aware of how people in wheelchairs feel and I can treat them with respect and sensitivity.

In Johannesburg there was another wheelchair and my bubble of joy started to evaporate. In Cape Town there was another wheelchair but this time my dear father was there and he did not treat me as if I was half alive. He showed such concern and sorrow for his sick and paralyzed daughter, and fussed over and coddled me.

The hospital felt strange and hostile and I started to feel my fear rising. I was so alone again. Maybe my father's fear had transmitted itself to me without my realizing it. I no longer had the support of my minister and believing friends who, although they thought I was euphoric, at least pandered to my faith by not openly doubting it. My dear father did not understand it at all and thought I was just being brave.

Dr Thorne was the first doctor to visit me and after listening to my account of the different attacks and reviewing the file I had brought down, and doing the usual prods, taps and pricks, said nothing and went to stand at the window looking out at Table Mountain. His silence made me nervous and uneasy.

"Well, Dr Thorne, what do you think?" I asked "Have I got multiple sclerosis or not?"

"I am sorry, my dear" he replied. "We will have to see what results the hospital comes up with but in my opinion after studying MS in England, yes, you have got multiple sclerosis."

All my fear returned and my faith plummeted to zero. I started to shake.

"What happens now?" I asked in a squeaky voice.

He shook his head. "I don't know. Nobody knows. This is the most unpredictable disease and no one knows what causes it, how it will progress or what will happen next."

In panic I almost shouted. "Does no one know anything about this disease?!"

He was quiet and looked briefly out of the window again then came slowly over to the bed.

"Yes," he said. "One person knows."

"Who is that?" I asked, thinking my father would take me anywhere for treatment.

Quietly with deep certainty the doctor replied. "God knows."

That was all I needed. God had spoken again. I lay back on the pillows exhausted and smiled tremulously at him. My faith was back.

"Thank you, doctor," I said. "I needed to hear that."

I am not sure Dr Thorne had faith in God's healing as he said no more. We didn't discuss it. I was too exhausted by then but God had used him. He could have meant that the disease was so unknown and unstudied that no one knew anything about it, but it did not matter to me.

My faith had returned and I turned over and fell asleep. When my faith was at its lowest ebb God had sent someone to tell me He was still there for me.

Of course, God knew all about this disease. He knew everything. I would just go to Him. He had already shown me by the anointing that He was the Healer and wanted to heal me so what was I afraid of? If God was for me, who could be against me?

The rest of my stay at Groote Schuur was much better. In my private room I read my bible and healing books and prayed. Several of the doctors saw the books by my bedside and looked at me enquiringly. I felt their attitude was one of pity. They pitied me for reading books like that. Some doctors, I have discovered, feel they have a monopoly on healing and God is left out of the equation.

They are almost insulted when you suggest God does the healing and they assist Him.

Some doctors, however, are becoming increasingly aware of the benefits of faith and hope for the healing of the body and their necessity for fighting any disease. They are a great encouragement to patients.

The sister in charge of my ward, Sister Peacock, was a Christian who believed in the divine intervention of God for healing and she was a great support to me. I knew she didn't have much faith for my healing, as she knew too much about the progression of multiple sclerosis, as she spoke to me about it. However she told me of the miracles in her life and that encouraged me. She would bring her cup of tea and we would talk of things of the Lord as if we had known each other forever. She was a real sister to me.

I had all the tests over again and got the terrible lumbar puncture headache. I had a mylogram and went blue on the table and had to be revived. I woke up from the anaesthetic with an oxygen mask over my face, and everyone crowding over me and rubbing my limbs looking scared. (Another miracle?) The devil couldn't get rid of me that quickly.

I could have been afraid then, as a doctor's hands are fallible, and they told me they were worried about my dying on the table. I did not even think about it until later. As far as I was concerned the doctors were in God's hands too.

Professor Aimes, the neurology professor, was a most interesting person and related to her patients like friends.

She did not talk down to me or hide anything from me. She told of the typical symptoms of MS, the stiff legged attempt at walking, the vibrations down your spine to under your feet when you put your chin on your chest. She explained that everything seemed to fit, but there was one thing that puzzled her about me.

"The one thing I can't understand about you," she said, "I don't understand why you are so peaceful and always smiling when most patients with MS are frightened, worried and depressed. I have never seen this before with MS. You are too happy!"

I was too happy!!!.

I tried to explain to her how God had shown me His love and presence in the anointing of heat, when Tony had prayed for me, and how this had taken away my fear. I knew I was in God's hands and He was healing me. I showed her the books I was reading and how God had confirmed everything to me in His word, the Bible.

I think she thought I was very strange. "Well," she said to me, "I still would like you to have an interview with the psychologist. There is something here which I do not understand and I want it checked out. Is that alright with you?"

"Just because I have faith that God is healing me, you think I am a psycho case?" I asked.

She smiled, "I just want it checked out."

Of course I had to agree but I knew this was an attack from evil powers trying to shake my faith and I had a spiritual battle on my hands. I was upset and angry. I prayed to get my peace back but I was not at ease when I went to see the psychiatrist. Psychologist or psychiatrist, whichever, I did not care. They were all the same to me and this felt like a witch hunt.

The psychiatrist started probing about my childhood and past experiences and was clearly surprised when I told him what excellent parents I had. Then he asked me about my marriage and I had to be honest and tell him about Malcolm's drinking problem which was a secret shame.

"Aha," he said. "This is it. You cannot cope with your marriage and have buried your problems. Your mind has engineered all these symptoms, subconsciously, so you can get attention. That is why you are so happy. You are now getting attention."

I was speechless with anger and indignation but what could I say? I tried to explain my faith but he was totally unreceptive. He just did not think that it was reasonable or logical for someone to trust God for healing and be happy and rest in this knowledge.

This psychiatrist probably did not believe there was a God at all, let alone a personal God who cared and loved His people enough to heal their physical sickness. His reality was not a healing God, but physical and mental illness that he could treat with psychoanalysis, electric shocks and drugs. I refused all of these.

The diagnosis from Groote Schuur was that if my illness was not psychological, it was Multiple Sclerosis.

I did not feel I could leave it that way and the day I was discharged I asked to see all the doctors and nurses. They crowded into my room, everyone from the professor to the cleaning ladies, to hear what this strangely happy young lady wanted to say to them. I told them about my experience of God's healing presence, the confirmation in His word, the Bible, and how it hurt that I was now considered unbalanced and a psychiatric case because I believed that God was healing me. I said I was happy because I knew God loved me, had touched me and was healing me although you couldn't yet see the healing.

Professor Aimes did apologize and say they had not meant to hurt me. Some of the nurses looked as if they believed me but on the whole I think the doctors thought this was just more evidence that I was unhinged. Hopefully if any of them read this book they will see that I was telling the truth.

After this, the headache from the lumber punctures got twice as bad and I had to delay my flight home and stay flat on my back until I recovered. My anger and emotion had caused a mini relapse. Now I could move even less and was back to square one. My dad had to dress and feed me again until I was well enough to fly back home.

But as I was lying there I remembered God's touch, His words of healing and saw again the pictures He had put in my mind. God is so good. He does not leave us alone.

I saw myself playing tennis again, running beside a stream on a farm and walking and working in my garden amongst the beautiful flowers and plants.

Psalm 20 v 7 says; Some may trust in horses,
Some may trust in chariots
But I will trust in the name of my God.

I was saying Some may trust in doctors,
Some may trust in medicine,
But I will trust in the name of my God.

My trip back to Zimbabwe was better. I was determined not to allow circumstances to destroy my faith again. There was a wheelchair waiting for me at Johannesburg airport but I pretended it was not for me. I hung on to the arm of a kind passenger instead. We arrived at the terminal 10 minutes after everyone else and my sister in law thought I had missed the plane. I battled walking, but I never used a wheelchair again.

Chapter 4

God's Airplane

When I got back to Gatooma the real work began.

If you go to a medical practitioner and he gives you medicine and treatment to follow, you do it all without question. I must do the same with my doctor, God.

1. God's first medicine was faith.
He had given me His faith when I had first felt the anointing of heat and healing, and I knew I must also walk in faith, doubting nothing, believing that I was healed. My doctor had all my trust and confidence. He was Almighty and Omniscient.

I had to take a dose of faith (more than a spoonful) through study of His word every day twice a day, morning and evening. I now knew how fragile human faith was, after my experience at Groote Schuur Hospital in Cape Town.

I could not let that happen again. The Bible says that faith comes by hearing and hearing from the word of God so I was going to steep myself in it.

I would also build up my faith by reading books by, and about people who had been healed by God. Tony raided his library and asked everyone for books for me. I started studying books by Andrew Murray and I still think his book 'Divine Healing' is the best on the subject.

I was sitting on the couch in my bedroom one day as usual, reading the gospel of John. I was thanking God for all the wonderful things in my life, my children, my loving husband and parents and then suddenly I saw a jumbo jet right before my eyes. It was so real I was astonished.

There it was, on a tarmac runway with neat cropped grass on either side. I had the feeling of space as there were no terminal buildings or hangars in my vision anywhere. It was just this enormous, white and silver plane on the runway in the middle of nowhere. It seemed shinier and bigger as there was nothing else to see.

I thought it must be because I had just been travelling by plane and I was puzzled, but then I heard a voice in my heart saying, "You must get onto that plane"

In my mind's eye, I saw myself running across the grass and tarmac and jumping eagerly up the stairs. I went in the doorway into the plane and it was empty. I thought this was strange but there was a warm secure feeling of peace and I was not afraid. I don't like crowds anyway and I felt special, as if this plane was exclusively for me.

I did not feel alone and felt as if I was floating in a lovely peaceful place. Then I heard the voice again telling me to sit down and buckle up my seat belt. I sat down and buckled up and saw the door close.
I felt safe and I heard the voice again. "You must climb into me as you have climbed into this plane. I, God, am your Airplane."

I was overwhelmed and excited. Did God say He was my Airplane in life? I absorbed this and thought about it and then said. "OK, God, that is wonderful and I receive that, but, Lord, where is Jesus?"

Immediately, the pilot stuck his head around the cabin door, smiled and gave me half a wave and half a salute. He looked so handsome in his pilot's cap, with dark eyes and hair and my heart thumped. He was so warm and friendly and I knew that the pilot of this plane was Jesus.

I relaxed in my seat while the engines started and we got ready for take off. However something was still puzzling me and I was feeling confident enough to ask.
So I said, "Thank you, Lord, and where is the Holy Spirit?"

The Lord replied; "The Holy Spirit is the air you need to breath as you fly. Without Him you cannot survive the altitude you will be flying at. Without Him you cannot live where I am taking you. You must always have the air of the

Holy Spirit moving in and out bringing My Life into your body. He must be as natural and present as breathing."

Now I knew just what to do and as the vision faded, the clarity of the message was all powerful. I had to climb into God and sit down, buckle up and relax as Jesus flew me to my destination and the Holy Spirit infused me with new healthy life. I couldn't do anything to help fly this plane. I couldn't do anything at all, except rest in God and get well.

I did not know where I was going but it did not matter at all. I was in the safest place of all. I could trust my pilot with my life, my way and my future. God was dependable, knew everything and loved me so much that He had put me in this place of complete security, in Him, in His Airplane.

I had just been reading John 15 again and I realized that God had given me my very own modern parable of this teaching. I had to remain in the vine and the sap of the Holy Spirit would come up into me and heal me and give me wonderful juicy bunches of grapes. The only pruning that God was doing to me and for me, was putting me into Himself, His Airplane, and keeping me sitting there buckled up so I couldn't get out. The door was closed and if I tried to get out I would die.

My independence, my will to do things my way, to think and do my own thing, was over and I felt a deep peace and inner joy. I had to live and have my being in Him completely and He was there always.

God's Airplane was to be my means of travel wherever I went in my life.

2. God's second medicine for me was exercise.
It was two years since I had played tennis and about one year since I had been able to walk at all so my muscles were weak. You can't expect God to get you walking again if your muscles are too weak to work. I had to prepare myself.

St Paul writes that he pressed on to win the race. All athletes train for the Olympic Games and I was in the biggest game of all; the game of life and death. It was biblical that I exercise my limbs so I could walk again when God healed me. I had to strengthen my body for that day.

I started doing exercises. The only exercises I could do were lying on the floor, so I lay on the floor and tried lifting my legs. It was a laugh and I managed to get them up about a centimetre and then collapsed exhausted but over the weeks this improved to about ten centimetres. I was making progress.

My cousins, Ian and Glynne, in Cape Town gave me a little book on hatha yoga. I didn't know anything about yoga and was not interested in the spiritual side, which I did not even know existed at this stage. I had my God and He was good. He had touched me and spoken to me so nothing else would get in the way.

The yoga exercises made sense though. I could only do slow stretching movements so it was ideal for me. The idea was to move your body to squeeze out the old blood and as you moved to a different position, new oxygenated blood filled that part. The deep breathing was obviously beneficial as fresh oxygen was necessary for healing.

God had told me that the Holy Spirit was the air I breathed in His Airplane so I concentrated on and thought of breathing in the life of the Holy Spirit. My exercise times became a special time with the Lord preparing my body for His use and breathing in His life-giving Spirit.

I knew that the brain and spinal cord were affected by MS so the inverted positions letting the blood flow to the brain must help, and the work stretching and moving the spine must be beneficial. I got there eventually. Everything was done so slowly that I could manage and I thought about God helping me with my 'workout'.

Gradually I became stronger and more supple. I always had to lie flat on the floor and rest for about half an hour afterwards but it was a warm comfortable place of complete relaxation. Slowly my body strengthened and I was able to do more.

I started to practise walking. First it was in the house, up and down the passage, leaning against the walls and then letting go for a few paces. When I felt more confident, I went out into the garden where I slowly walked around hanging on to the trees.

At last I determined to walk around the block.

I never told anyone where I was going as everyone had been given strict instructions by the doctor that they must see that I rested and did nothing. I just slipped away silently one morning when Joy was sleeping and the boys were at school.

There was bravado and determination in my heart and I started confidently enough, hanging onto the fence and dragging myself along the unkempt grass pavement under the huge Msasa trees. Then there was a wall to lean on and I literally pulled myself along.

I thought I was doing well until I was about half way. I was absolutely exhausted, my legs felt like jelly, I was dizzy and could not take another step. There was a rock nearby and I crawled to it and sat down to take stock.

Had I climbed out of my Airplane? Was I doing my own thing again? I hadn't actually asked the Lord if I should do this. Maybe I was stepping out on my own, in my own strength. No wonder I was feeling so ill. God had told me I could do nothing without Him.

I prayed. "Sorry, Lord for going my own way and not consulting You first. I am sure learning my lesson. Please God get me home"
I felt calmer but still too ill and weak to move.

Should I go back or trust that I would make the round trip? I was so sorry now that I had not told the nanny where I was going. She would have sent someone to look for me. I decided that it was as far to go back as to go forward, so I may as well go on. I would complete the task I had set myself.

I gritted my teeth and pulled myself up on the fence and dragged myself on. Now it was much slower, every step an effort. I willed my legs to move, praying all the time. "God, please help me. Lord, I'm sorry I did this without asking you. Lord Jesus, please get me home."

The last little way was too much. There was no one around as we lived in a very quiet suburb with large properties and everyone was at work. I hung on to that fence for dear life, my legs wobbly and refusing to move another inch.

I was close to home now and I could see the garden. Hopefully the gardener would be within range and I called as loudly as I could. Thank God, he heard me and came running to almost carry me home.

I had made it, but not on my own. My Jumbo Jet got me home and I learned another lesson. After that, I never attempted anything without asking the Lord first. It was God who had helped me, as I had been at the end of my own strength.

Malcolm offered to sell the car and buy an automatic so I could drive. Several people offered to buy me a wheelchair at a really good price but I refused them all. To do this would be to admit defeat and this I refused to do. I was being healed and I would walk and drive normally again.

From then on I got stronger and stronger. I was still doing my exercises every day and was quite pleased with my progress. A couple of months later I started driving the car and then after a few more months was able to do a bit of slow shopping.

A Jewish friend of mine, Leslie, stopped me once in a shop;
"You look so beautiful and happy," she said. "It is as if there is a light shining from you."
I was amazed that people could actually see what God was doing to me and in me.
"Thank you," I replied. "It is the touch of God. He is healing me."
At last I even managed to play the organ in church again but they still went on praying for me.

3. The third medicine God showed me was nutrition.
The first book I got hold of was by Adelle Davis 'Lets Get Well' and it struck a chord in my spirit.

God made us. He made us in His own image and He made us well and healthy. He looked at all He had made, and said it was good so He didn't make us to be sick. He gave us dominion over every plant and food so He gave us the where-with-all to look after our bodies and remain healthy. Therefore we must adopt His wisdom and use every plant and food to get healthy again if we are sick.

The first thing I learnt was that vitamin B was most important for nerve function and in MS the nerves and the myelin sheath are attacked by the body's own immune system. If you have MS you get little holes in the myelin sheath and the exposed nerves get tangled and lead to all the funny sensations and abnormalities we feel. Sometimes these exposed nerves die, leading to paralysis and loss of bodily functions. Sometimes these little holes heal over again and the nerves recover or another part of the brain takes over the impaired function.

I was sure that God would heal over my little holes and bring back all my normal functions and I would use God's every source of nutrition to help.

I started taking 10 brewers yeast tablets three times a day, this being the best source of vitamin B at that time. I started giving myself Vitamin B injections once a week and this regimen really helped my energy levels, and I could go on longer without the complete exhaustion, when it was an effort to hold my head up.

I tried taking lecithin as the myelin sheath is made up of this, but I was allergic to that and came out in bumps all over my body. It was a matter of trial and error.I started eating sunflower seeds like a parrot and would nibble them whenever I felt like a snack. I still do.

Later on I took Evening Primrose oil capsules. Professor Reef at the Johannesburg General Hospital told me, that all this would do, was keep me young, but I thought this alone was an excellent reason for taking it. I know it has helped as when I have gone off it I have felt a slight regression. Nothing is immediate as natural remedies take time to work, but you do notice the difference over time.

I still took the cortisone which my human doctor prescribed, but when he put me onto ACTH injections (synthetic cortisone) I once again came out in bumps and had to stop. Later I was given Immuran, potassium and amitryptiline by the doctors and I took it all but I don't know how well it worked.It did not matter as God was healing me, not the cortisone, injections or tablets but as God also uses doctors, I never refused the treatment and did what I was told.

4. The fourth medicine God gave me was prayer.
I had to remain in my Airplane and communicate constantly with the Holy Spirit breathing into me. Communication involves not only talking but more importantly listening. I learned to listen to God, keeping my spiritual ears open particularly when I was reading the word.

I also learned to listen to my body. When I was tired, I had to lie down and rest and then God talked to me. Often I would fall asleep with one of the beautiful pictures He gave me of resting in His arms in a cloud.

When I was in pain, however, God gave me the vision of His powerful laser beam shining down on me and cutting out the pain. He showed me how to embrace all the magnificence of the stars and the universe in my mind, and gather it into one shining beam coming down to me.

God's creation is so vast, we have to stretch our minds to fathom it, but as we practise seeing the wonder of His universe, we can gather that awesome power into a beam in our imagination. We can, in our mind's eye, see it coming down to ourselves for healing and cutting out pain and illness. After the pain in my neck was healed by God in the initial prayer, I didn't have much pain over the years, but I know that some MS sufferers have a lot of pain. Cancer sufferers also have a great deal of pain and this exercise will help them. I called it my 'prayer for pain exercise'.

God taught me to see His healing in that beam of light. There would be warmth and comfort, the pain would go and I would sleep. This became an invaluable action to remove any pain I suffered and I would recommend it for anyone. The mental concentration required is quite intense, but it is worth the effort, and allows God's healing right into the afflicted area to remove pain. I would see this beam of God healing over the little holes in my myelin sheath and cutting out any area of sickness.

5. However the greatest medicine that God showed me was His Word.
Above all, I studied the Word and learned all He had to say about healing. I couldn't accept my healing only with blind faith, based on the wonderful experience of the heat of God flowing through me. I had to reason it all out and understand with my head as well as my heart.

I wrote it all down; every scripture where God promised to heal, and every healing miracle of Jesus. God is the same yesterday, today and forever (Hebrews 13.8) and as Jesus was God come down to earth, and He lived only to do the will of the Father, then He was doing the Father's will to heal.

Therefore it is God's will to heal.

Chapter Five

What God Says

I wanted to know everything my doctor, God, had to say and He talks to us through His Word, the Bible.

As I wrote down all the scriptures on healing, I started analyzing them and putting together the meaning for me.

The first thing I saw was that God was good.

Right from Genesis to Revelations the theme of God's word is that He is a good God, He made us, He loves us, and He only wants to bless us. I had known the Lord from a little girl but I really had to let the **goodness** of God sink into my heart and mind in a new way.

Jeremiah 29:11 says. "I know the plans I have for you," says the Lord, "plans for your welfare and not for evil, to give you a future and a hope."

If He wanted only my welfare, then sickness was not in His plan, He did not bring it on me and healing and wholeness was what He wanted for me. He wanted to give me a future and a hope, and suffering from a paralyzing disease was no future to look forward to. I did not want that but neither did my good God.

Where then did sickness come from? If God rules and reigns how can sickness come to torment us?

The thing is that man has rejected God's rule and is just interested in doing his own thing so evil (or the devil) actually rules on earth through man.

Jesus said "The thief comes only to steal, kill and destroy; I came that they may have life and life abundantly." (John10;10)

Sickness is not abundant life, and it is the devil, the evil thief, that steals, kills and destroys and brings sickness. We have given Satan authority by rejecting the rule of God. I knew these basics but they became much more real and personal to me now that Satan had stolen my health.

In Luke 13:11-17 we read the story of Jesus healing the woman who was bent over. Jesus said the woman had been bound by **Satan** for 18 years and He healed her.

Therefore Satan brings sickness and God heals and releases from the oppression of evil. Sickness is evil not good. God saves from evil and its consequences. Jesus died on the cross to save us from sin, Satan and oppression of evil including sickness. By His stripes we are healed. Isaiah 53:4-5

It is not true that God brings sickness to punish people. Satan can get at God only through us, so he wants us to suffer to hurt God. It is Satan who brings sickness.

Does God want to heal?
Some people seem to think that it is God's will that they are sick, and I had to sort this out in my own mind, as I didn't want to go against God's will. After studying all the scriptures I realized this line of thinking was maligning the character of God.

The bible says God loves us and that He is love. If it is His word then it is God talking to us. He says He is LOVE. He made us in His image and our parental love, therefore, comes from Him. Our love is imperfect and much inferior to His, but we don't want our children sick. We do all in our power to make them better. So why would our Heavenly Father want His children to be sick? It is an insult to Him to think that way.

When did Jesus ever refuse to heal anyone who asked Him?
Matthew 8;1-3 He tells the leper He **wants** to heal him and He does.
Matthew 8;7 He tells the centurion He **will** come and heal his sick servant.
Mark5;22 He **does not hesitate** to go with Jairus to heal his daughter.

Luke 13;11-13 Jesus **calls** the woman to come to Him and then He heals her.

I could go on and on. It is all there in the stories of Jesus.

The closest Jesus ever got to refusing healing was with the Syrophoenician woman who asked him to heal her daughter. She was a pagan, who did not believe in God, but when she showed that she believed, He healed her daughter. Mark 7:24-30

Also Jesus did not heal everyone at the pool, but they were all looking to the pool to heal them, and did not ask Him. (John 5:2-8). The pool could be an allegory of people looking to human doctors **only**, or people looking to **false gods**, and not to Jesus for healing. God often works with human doctors to heal.

We have to believe in a good God and in what Jesus did for us. We have to believe He is almighty, and wants to heal us and that sickness is not brought by Him.

We also have to believe that Jesus can heal at a distance, as He did for the Syrophoenician woman and the centurion's servant. We cannot see Him now but He is here by His Spirit, and if He healed at a distance when He walked this earth, of course He can heal now, when He is seated at the right hand of the Father and working by His Spirit here on earth. The Holy Spirit is with us.

Jesus healed with compassion. God has compassion for His people. Whatever I was going through and whatever you are going through, God understands and has compassion. He walked this earth so He knows what life is like here. He is not light years away looking down at us with a microscope. He is here with us in a spirit of compassion.

I had to understand thoroughly that God knew all about me, knew about my disease, had compassion and wanted to heal. I had to realise that He was with me always and I had to get into Him like the Airplane He showed me.

I had to internalize the fact that He is willing and able to do far more abundantly than all I could ask or think. Ephesians 3:20. If this is the case then, of course, He was willing and able to heal me.

I had to **resist** any doubt or fear that the devil brought on me. James 4:7.
I had to realize that if God was **for** me, who could be against me. Romans 8:31.
I had to **abide** in Jesus, **rest** in Him and then I could not help but be healed. John 15:4
I had to **live** in Him, **move** in Him and **have my being** in Him, Acts 17:27 and He would be healing me all the time.
It had to be no longer I that lived but **Christ who lived in me**. Galations 2:20

I used my mind and imagination to picture myself in Jesus and He in me, not only in the Airplane but also as a body and a person. I had to be like a glove sandwiched between Jesus within and Jesus on the outside. He was like a protective space suit I was wearing but He was also within

48

me. I must be like a living container, a Christ container, holding Him inside me.

Also everyday I had to put on the full armour of God, which is putting on Jesus. He is our Truth, our Righteousness, our Prince of Peace, our Salvation and the Word of God. Ephesians 6:10-18.

I read all these scriptures, learnt them, repeated them, and praised and thanked God for them and my healing, and so I gradually got better.

Whenever I got depressed, fell, or lost control of my emotions (tears or temper which are very prevalent with MS) I would go back to that quiet place of peace in God; into His Airplane where His peace enfolded me and the healing could continue.

I learned I had to pray without ceasing. God's word told me it was part of His armour, so I must do it.
At first I found this totally daunting. How could I pray all the time when I had three children, a husband to care for, a home to run, and I was sick and everything I did was an effort anyway?

I had been blessed with a very understanding husband and two wonderful servants in the house, but I still had to organize and supervise and give my children loving attention.

I learnt that praying without ceasing was to remain in God's presence, chat to Him and refer everything to Him all the time. I asked Him what we should have for dinner and what the children could be doing to keep them occupied and what I should be doing in the house.

At first I thought this was ridiculous and He couldn't be interested in these little decisions in my day, but I saw that if I was to remain in His presence, and pray without ceasing, this is what He wanted. I also had to thank Him constantly for all the good things in my life, the flowers, trees and beautiful world around us and every little improvement in my health.

I studied all His promises for prayer and I was so determined to get my healing and wanted Him to heal me so much, that I learned with joy that He said He was far more ready to listen than we are to pray.

I learned that Jesus said "Whatever you ask in my name, I will do it so that the Father may be glorified in the Son: If you ask anything in my name, I will do it." John 14:12

In biblical language 'in His name' means so much more than today. It means in Christ's character, in His very self, all that He stands for, and He stands for goodness, love and healing. This meant that I could ask and expect Him to do anything He would have done when He was on earth, and He healed here on earth.

Jesus also said in John 15:7, "If you abide in me and my words abide in you, ask whatever you will and it shall be done for you." This scripture really excited me as He had already told me that I must abide in Him, get into Him as an Airplane, sit down and buckle up so He could fly me where He wanted me to go.

I could therefore expect Him to heal me. He said so, so it must be so. He would answer my prayer for healing.

In Matthew 21:22 and Mark 11:24 Jesus also said "Whatever you ask in prayer, you will receive it if you have faith" and "Whatever you ask in prayer believe that you receive it and you will."

He had given me the gift of faith, and now all that I studied and read, built up that faith, as I continued in His presence. He also gave me the pictures of running, walking and playing with the children when I was healed, and this meant I SAW my healing, which is faith.

1 John 5:14 says; "and this is the confidence we have in Him, that if we ask anything according to His will, He will hear us. And if we know He hears us in whatever we ask, we know we have obtained the requests made of Him"

I had already established that God had not brought my sickness, that He had saved us from sickness on the cross, and that it was His will to heal, so I knew I was asking in His will.

God also gave me techniques of how to pray, particularly when I was lying down and resting, which was very often at the beginning.

I would lie down and see myself on a cloud, a cloud of God's glory, holding me, cuddling me and penetrating my body as He healed me. 'Underneath are the everlasting arms.'

I would see myself sitting on Jesus' lap like a little child. "Suffer the little children to come unto me." He said. (Matthew 19:13-15)

I would see myself lying beside the 'still waters' in beautiful surroundings just enjoying the beauty of His creation, and His peace and healing would flow into me. Psalm 23.

As I said before, I would see myself under the stars, and greater than that, the enormity of the whole universe, which I could not even fathom. His power would flow down to me in a beam of light, power and heat which infused my body with His healing and took away my pain. 'How great are your mighty works O God.' Psalm 19.

I would see myself running and playing with my children and even playing tennis again. "Those that wait upon the Lord shall mount up like eagles, they shall run and not be weary, they shall walk and not faint." Isaiah 40:31

So I personalized these scriptures and I put any of these pictures in my mind when I was resting and praying, sitting in His Airplane, and it all came to pass. It happened just as Jesus said.

About five years later I went back onto the tennis court to knock a couple of balls.

Chapter Six

War and Prayer

Malcolm at last found a farm that he wanted to buy and we moved to Fort Victoria (now Masvingo). We looked over the rolling valley to the hills in the east and fell in love with the farm.

It was a beautiful farm in the Happy Valley. The homestead was on a hill overlooking our irrigated lands and we could just see the buildings of Bikita Minerals in the distance. In the south was a single hill, called Mara, meaning impala, in Shona. We had a big dam on the stream bordering the Gutu Reserve and water was pumped up to a storage dam above the lands and led by gravity to irrigate the crops. For a family picnic, there was another uncultivated valley behind the house where a little stream ran. In the paddock beside the house, were two old horses and plenty of room for cattle and more horses.

I was happy to go, as there was hope in Malcolm's eyes. His vision had always been for a successful crop farm, and I did so want this for him. However I was separated from my church, friends and more importantly my minister, who was feeding my faith and helping every step of the way in my healing.

It was lovely living on a farm again but we had to put our eldest son, Kenneth, in boarding school although he was only seven. He didn't cry, but mother did. I then home-schooled our second son Douglas with 'School on the Air' and it was a wonderful bonding time for us. Joy was only a little thing but she joined in and later I home-schooled her too.

I had plenty of time to be with the Lord and the quietness of the country was a balm for the soul.
Then I had another MS attack and I was devastated. I knew God was healing me and I had been so well. I was walking and gardening a little and even learning to ride the horses and now this! It was not as severe as before, but I immediately phoned Tony who put me in touch with the Methodist minister in Fort Victoria.

Peter was a gentle, kindly young man and he drove the 60 miles out to the farm to see me. We sat and chatted and I told him my story and a bit about MS, as he didn't know anything about the disease. Then he proceeded to quote Psalm 22 (the psalm Jesus quoted on the cross) and say that maybe I was called to suffer for the Lord.

I was so angry as this was exactly opposite what God had shown me in His word. MS sufferers will know how volatile one's emotions are in an attack and how swiftly the blood boils. I said nothing but started shaking, and reached for my Bible to find this psalm. I would see for myself what God said to me.

In my lap, the Bible fell open to Psalm 103 and the words jumped out at me bold and blacker than all the other writing on the page.

> **Bless the Lord, O my soul; and all that is within me, bless his holy name!**
> **Bless the Lord, O my soul, and forget not all his benefits,**
> **Who forgives all your iniquity, and heals all your diseases.**

I was so amazed I started to laugh with relief.

Peter was puzzled. He had told me I was to suffer for the Lord and now I was laughing. When I showed him and read it to him, he laughed ruefully and agreed that this was truly a promise from the Lord, that I would be healed.
We parted great friends but he had instilled a niggling doubt in me.

I had been to the Anglican Church in Fort Victoria but I was craving something a bit more lively, so when I got well enough to drive, I bundled the kids into the car and we headed for the Full Gospel church in town. I was not very impressed by the preacher as he jumped about the platform, and I was not used to that, however at the end of the service, he stood still and was silent a while. Then he said that the Lord had just told him that there was someone here, with an incurable disease and that this person must come up for prayer.

My hair stood on end. I couldn't believe it, I was so amazed.

I had never been into a church where this sort of thing happened, but I immediately put Joy down from my lap and went to the front. There was no way that preacher could know anything about me, as we had only just moved into the area and I knew no one.

This time there were no sensations of heat, but I knew by that word of knowledge from the preacher, that God had heard my prayers to heal me. I was being healed and Psalm 22 was not for me.

The children and I sang choruses all the way home.

I phoned Tony in excitement, and told him all about it and he said that strange things were also happening in Gatooma, and people were talking in tongues.
"Oh no," I said. "You don't have to be weird and emotional to be a Christian. That sounds like nonsense to me."
"Well," he replied, "I'll send you some books."
"OK" I said. "I am never averse to reading up on things."

The books arrived the next week and once I started reading, I couldn't stop. I read 'Nine o'clock in the Morning' by Dennis Bennet, 'Prison to Praise' by Merlin Caruthers, and 'They Spoke with Other Tongues.' By John Sherrill. At the end I said, "Lord, I want it too."

I was telling our farm manager and his wife all about it. Their cousin from a mission station on the other side of Fort Victoria happened to be visiting and she said very casually. "Oh the people, who have been praying for others to speak in tongues, have just been to our mission station but left this morning and won't be back for another month or so."

"Please can you let me know when they come back so I can come over?" I asked.

"Sure" she said.

I went home happy that I would also have the Baptism of the Holy Spirit in a couple of months.

She phoned me next day and said these people were back unexpectedly, and they didn't know why.

I said silently in my heart, 'Lord you are rushing me.'

"Go" said the quiet voice and I was reminded that Jesus said "He that puts his hand to the plough and turns back, is not worthy"

I went. I bundled Douglas and Joy into the car and we drove the 120miles to the mission station on the other side of town.

When I got there I was astounded to see that these were youngsters of about 18 and 19. They were with YWAM. (Youth with a Mission). I expected someone older and more responsible and was immediately very wary. When they questioned me to find out if I had given my heart to the Lord, I was quite offended.

I had been a Christian a long time, long before they were born. If I hadn't driven such a long way to get this 'Baptism in the Holy Spirit' I would probably have left, but I swallowed my pride and answered all their questions satisfactorily.

They prayed for me and immediately light flooded down on me. I was the only one who saw it but it was so real.

This was not heat, like when Tony had prayed for my healing, but light, a great bright light streaming down from heaven, beaming on me and around me like a cone. I think now, that it must have been something like the light that converted and blinded Saul. It was amazing and wonderful. I just knelt there basking in it.

Then they started praying in tongues and told me to open my mouth and start doing it too. Well I opened my mouth and started praying in English.
"No," they said, "not in English. Let your tongue loose and let God speak through you."

Well, I tried but I couldn't. Maybe I was too self conscious. Maybe I refused to give up my control of myself. Maybe because I thought 'tongues' was weird I subconsciously refused. Whatever the reason, I couldn't do it and they struggled with me for quite a while, until I called a halt and said I must start on the long drive back home.

I knew, however, that I had been filled by the Holy Spirit because of that light, and a new joy that bubbled in my heart. It felt as if God held me on an elastic band. Whenever I got too far from abiding in the Lord, and the elastic band stretched, I felt it pull and was tugged back with a powerful force. I walked in the hills above the farmstead and practiced talking in tongues among the Msasa trees. I managed a few words and now I speak fluently, as long as I do not listen to myself, as then I get tongue-tied. I now use it to pray for others when I do not know what to pray.

I had MS attacks on the farm but they got milder and less frequent. I continued with my exercises and my resting in the Lord. Whereas MS usually goes downhill like a staircase, with attacks coming and going making the body progressively weaker, mine was like walking up a staircase. I was getting better and better after attacks and my body was getting stronger all the time.

The doctor in Fort Victoria put me on cortisone again but I gained an enormous amount of weight, so after a couple of months we stopped it and I went on just with my vitamins, exercises, and resting in my Airplane with the Lord.

The children were wonderful to me when I was ill. I am so ashamed looking back, at the swift bursts of temper I suffered from. The children learned to handle them before I did. They would take me by the hand and gently lead me to bed.

"Come, Mommy, you are sick," they would say. "You need to lie down. We will get you a nice cup of tea."

The first time they did this, I burst into tears. Out of the mouths of babes.

Later they just had to say that I needed to lie down, and I would smile and my anger subsided. Then I did learn to control it and when I felt anger rising, would go and lie down on my own until I was feeling better. I would lie down and release all my tension in the cloud, held by the 'everlasting arms', and come into the Lord's presence beside the 'still waters'.

The children were also so caring when I was battling to walk. We went as a family to the Zimbabwe Ruins and when I couldn't get up the hill to the acropolis, they took turns pushing me from behind. It was hilarious and other tourists must have thought we were so silly but we turned a disability into a game. I got there laughing and the children loved it.

I taught myself to play the guitar and started a morning prayer and song session with the maids on the farm. It started in the kitchen but as more people wanted to join, we went down to the sheds. What a lovely time of praise and worship we had. I learned the guitar from books my parents sent me, so I played very badly but no one cared. We had fun and blessings, singing and praising the Lord.

I am not sure if any of them came to the Lord as I was very amateurish in my preaching. All I told them was how wonderful God was, and how He loved them, just where they were. They changed and became a happy crowd, singing spiritual songs as they went about their work.

Then they started bringing their sick children to me and I would dress cuts and wounds, attend to sick tummies and sore chests and pray for them. At least they knew that I loved the Lord and was doing what I could for them. No one refused the prayer so I am sure God touched them even if I couldn't speak their language.

I had plenty of time for quiet with the Lord and I was at peace. Malcolm was busy on the farm working so hard, that he didn't have time for drinking much, so we had peace in the home as well.

My dear cousin Percival, who is more like a brother to me, wrote that he had become a Christian and I was so thrilled. I wrote back saying I was also a committed Christian. I was dismayed when I received a reply to the effect that, there was no such thing as a committed Christian, only a born again one, and that if I hadn't been baptized by full immersion, it was not the real thing.

Once again I was upset but I love the stimulation of a good discussion.

I got out my concordance and all the different versions of the Bible and set out to do a Bible study to see if he was right. I discovered that 'born again' was the terminology for asking Jesus to take over your life, so I was obviously born again, but I hadn't been baptized by total immersion. Although I saw that this did not mean I was not saved, it is a command of Jesus, and I felt I must have this done. I wanted to do everything He told me to do.

I went to a little church in Fort Victoria, the Apostolic Faith Mission, where my friend Alice van Heerden worshipped, and asked the pastor to baptize me. The whole family came to support me although Malcolm thought it was very strange. It was a good experience for me, as I knew I was acting in obedience to the Lord, identifying with Him in death and resurrection.

When I told the Anglican minister what I had done, I was shocked when he told me I was excommunicated from the church. I loved my church where I had worshipped all my life, played the organ and where they had prayed for me so faithfully. I wrote to the bishop in Salisbury (Harare) and had such a gracious reply that if the Lord had so obviously told me to be baptized by total immersion then I was right to do so and I was not excommunicated.

The war broke out in the country in 1966. We never had legislated apartheid in Rhodesia but there was segregation of blacks and whites and the blacks did not have a vote or a say in government. Now the Matabele and Shona People formed political parties, went for military training outside the country and took up arms against the whites. Their soldiers moved into the rural areas and the farmers and rural blacks were their targets. They attacked and killed indiscriminately and we were all vulnerable and afraid. The farm workers were terrified as, if they cooperated with us they were attacked and maimed or killed.

Soon the war came to our region as well and we joined the police reserve to protect ourselves. I was quite a crack shot on the rifle range but the only time I had to shoot at an intruder, I shot and fainted. The man was circling our house at dawn and did not stop when hailed. He ran up into the hill and was almost out of sight so this was just a warning shot but the shooting was too much for me. Shooting at a person, however far away, was very different to shooting at a target. My head spun and I fell in a dead faint. I would never have made a soldier

After this, the government put up security fences around the house and gave us an agric- alert radio.

Kenneth drove the mini-moke on the farm and learnt to shoot by the time he was 11. We would travel into town with a 38 special revolver on my lap, an uzi issued by the police reserve, next to me, and the shot gun, which Kenneth held. A couple of our neighbours were attacked on the way to town and we were taking no chances, but we knew it was God who protected us.

If we went on a drive or a picnic in the back valley of the farm, we went well armed and even little Joy carried the .22 by the time she was 7. We learned to live with it, but it was not pleasant.

We saw our neighbours, the Nolans, at the top of the valley shot up and sat on our veranda shivering and praying while the agric-alert crackled, mortars flew and the gun shots resounded. Malcolm was told not to go in and help but to stay with his family, as the troops were on their way. As quickly as the attack started it stopped. Their house was partly burned down and one of the sons and the mother were wounded, but they got off lightly.

Another neighbour was ambushed on his way to town and both he and his wife were wounded but he fired back and killed one of the attackers. I prayed that this would never happen to us. We started staggering our trips into town so they would not know our schedule. We knew they were there in the hills watching us.

Our neighbours on the other side of the Mara Hill were attacked and their house burnt down. We saw the glow of the fire above the hill and heard the gunfire and explosions of the mortars. They were older folk and never recovered from the shock. They lost everything and moved away, back to England.

The casual, friendly atmosphere on the farm changed to one of nervous tension. We still got on very well with our labour force, and I still had the praise song sessions at the sheds, but Malcolm carried a gun wherever he went, and the children stayed behind the fence all the time, unless they were with us.

I grew even closer to God at this time as I spent so much time with Him.
One day when I was spending time praying for the country, God gave me a distinct message that the country as a whole must pray, and I must mobilize them.

I was terrified. Oh no, what could I, a little insignificant farmers wife, do to get the country praying? I put the thought out of my mind.

Our farm was situated on the boundary of the Gutu Reserve which was heavily infiltrated by the freedom fighters. We called them 'terrs' and they committed dreadful atrocities against their own people. It was a terrible war with atrocities on both sides and most of the time the farmers were in the middle.

We had to do something, but God was the only one who could sort this out. There were Christians on both sides of the conflict and I did not feel it was right to pray for victory for either side. We needed God's solution. The idea of getting the whole country praying persisted and wouldn't leave me alone.

Eventually I said to God, "Alright, Lord if you want me to do this, then you must please give me help, as I cannot do this on my own. If you provide a partner for me, then I will know that this is of You, that it is Your will and I must do it. Please give me assurance and clear direction."

I was so frightened and with my knees knocking, I stood up at the next Agricultural Union meeting and said that the Lord had called us all to pray. They agreed and several people said that they were praying; parliament always started with a prayer, and their churches were praying, but no one came forward to offer any help. I relaxed and thought that I had imagined everything and I did not have to do anything else but pray myself.

Next day I had to phone the accountant where my friend, Alice, worked. I generally had to ask the receptionist to put me through when I wanted to talk to her. On this day, however, she answered the phone herself, and I was surprised and pleased to have the opportunity to chat, before being put through to our accountant. We spoke for a while and then I mentioned that God was telling me that we must all as a nation, all races together, pray for the country.

"Yes," she said. "You are quite right. The Lord has been speaking to me about that as well, but it is such an enormous undertaking."

"Would you help me of you felt the Lord wanted us to do this?" I asked tentatively. "I have felt the Lord urging me forward, but I cannot do it alone. I have asked Him to give me a partner if He wants me to do this. Then I will know it is His will."

"OK" she said. "I will pray about it tonight and let you know tomorrow."

I left it in God's hands and next day she phoned and said she would do it, but like a true accountant, she added that it must not cost us any money as neither of us had anything and we couldn't get into debt.

I hadn't even thought of the money, but I agreed and said that if this was what God wanted from us, He would supply our needs.

We met and with prayer decided on a strategy. We would have a prayer printed on a pamphlet in English, Shona and Ndebele and would spread them around the whole country through the churches. We would choose a day when all the churches would pray together, and we would put out bumper stickers and posters that all the churches would give to their members to use, give to others and put up the posters.

We would also contact parliament and the radio stations so that this prayer would be prayed at noon. We would call it 'The Pray for Rhodesia Campaign' and print our address at the bottom, so if anyone wanted to help us they knew where to find us.

Now we had to find the right prayer and with much prayer of our own, we finally came up with;

Lord, Bless our country,
May your will be done
And show me how to do my part.

We reasoned that the blessing of God meant peace, stability and prosperity so all that was included in the prayer. We wanted a short prayer that everyone could remember, and we did not want any one side promoting it for their own ends. We knew that God's will was the only solution and each person must seek God's will for himself/herself.

I went to the local printer in Fort Victoria to have the pamphlets printed and there they were translated into Shona and Ndebele. They gave us a special price and I chose the cheapest paper but was still astonished at the cost of it all. I phoned all the churches and alerted them to what we were doing, asking how many pamphlets they needed and getting their cooperation to give them out, but I never asked for money.

We designed a logo, car stickers and posters with the map of Rhodesia in green overlaid with a brown cross and red writing. The pamphlets were only black and white with a small logo so there was no doubt that we were praying through the cross, in Jesus' name.

Then the money started coming in, from churches and individuals who had heard we were doing this by faith. We could pay the phone bill, the printer's bill and petrol costs, and we started posting packets of pamphlets to all the churches. Alice came over, I roped in my family and we made parcel after parcel, piled them into the cars and filled the post office counter to overflowing. It was a busy but exciting time.

When we had finished, the only amount outstanding was $600 for the posters and that came in from a single supporter at a prayer group in Harare (Salisbury). God is good. He undertook completely. The whole campaign cost about $30000 which was a great deal of money at that time and we didn't have to pay for anything ourselves. . Malcolm looked on in amazement when the money came in, and all our costs were paid. God had provided for His work.

The day of prayer went off with gusto and the newspapers reported that everyone was praying. The radio went on using the prayer at noon for a couple of months and we could feel a lifting of the desperation in so many people as they turned to God for help.

Maybe we did not pray specifically enough, maybe we did not pray long enough or go on praying and only God knows the reason Zimbabwe turned out as it did. The country and the government turned away from the Lord. Christians were being persecuted and poverty, sickness and suffering are still so widespread it is a dreadful tragedy.

We can just pray that the new government and the country will again turn to the Lord and be saved. Many of the poor, I know love and serve the Lord and there are still vibrant churches but if they did not support the old government they were persecuted and their pastors attacked, their homes burnt down and their families in some cases even killed..

During this time of frenetic activity, visiting printers and designers, travelling to and from Harare, visiting ministers and pastors, speaking at meetings etc., I never had one symptom of MS. No spiders or ants or cramps, no loss of feeling or trouble with walking. God kept me absolutely well while I was doing His work.

After a couple of months, when it was all completed, I even went back to the tennis court for my first short game. It was so exciting to have my vision fulfilled after five long years even if I could only hit a couple of balls to start with.

Chapter 7

Reconciliation in Death

We received so many letters of appreciation that, I am afraid, I started thinking what a good job we had done. Yes, the Lord had prompted it and done it, but as His instruments, we had done well. Perhaps I became smug and proud but whatever the reason I was not aware of the storm clouds gathering.

It could be that Satan was fed up with our prayer campaign and organized an attack that would stop us and remove me from Rhodesia completely.

We lost the farm.
We never recovered from the drought of the first year and Malcolm borrowed an enormous amount of money to concrete the irrigation canals for irrigation for the next year, but we had floods; 7 inches of rain the first year and 45 the next. We planted maize the first year and it died

in the drought. We planted cotton the next year as it is drought resistant, but in the flood year the cotton rotted and we lost that as well.

After battling with the enormous debt for a couple of years, we went into judicial management to try and save something. The executors put a manager on the farm and Malcolm got a job at Mkwasine in the Lowveld, as a section manager in the winter wheat growing section.

This was a major disaster. Devastated at losing the farm, Malcolm started drinking from morning to night. In fact he was drunk by breakfast time. I roped the children in to help look for the hidden bottles but as fast as we threw them out, so he bought more and found new hiding places.

The war activities were also closer here. We heard people walking past our security fence one night and discovered next morning that one of the mechanics, Pinto, had been abducted and marched right next to our house on his way to Mozambique. The army lost track of him over the border and he was never seen again. It was a scary time and while I prayed more, Malcolm drank more.

All three children were at boarding school in Fort Victoria and we had to travel to and fro in convoy protected by troops and a helicopter. We actually saw the freedom fighters on a few occasions, on top of the hills in the pass. Once our convoy was attacked and one of the civilians and a couple of troops were killed when a mortar hit them. It all happened behind us at the end of the convoy, so we were not directly involved, but it was a nasty experience nevertheless.

Our children were being badly affected by Malcolm's constant drinking. Although he was an amiable drunk and would just slur his words, be stupid and fall down, we were all deeply ashamed of his behaviour and the stigma associated with it.

Looking for the bottles of alcohol was a constant horror and tension, but we would try to laugh together at the ridiculous places we found them; in the toilet cistern, on top of the pelmets, in his boots and even in the chicken run in the nesting boxes, amongst the newly laid eggs.

Obviously people thought we were tarred with the same brush so they started avoiding us and we shrank into ourselves. I would take the children down to swim in the estate swimming pool, when I was sure there would be no one else there, and I made no friends. The nearest church was in Chiredzi, too far to drive on my own. Anyway I didn't want to see anyone, or talk to anyone. I just wanted to hide in a corner and lick my wounds.

Malcolm lost his job at Mkwasine because of the drinking and went on a three-month stint to the border with the police reserve. I put the furniture into storage and got a job, as a matron, at the Andrew Louw School outside Fort Victoria, while the children were at the government school in town. I was very happy as a matron, tending all the minor illnesses, cuts and bruises, playing my guitar and singing and praying with the children before they went to sleep.

I took stock of my life and decided to leave Malcolm and make a new life for myself and my children in Cape Town with my parents. When Malcolm came out of police reserve, I went to meet him in Chiredzi to tell him.

I re-established contact with the Methodist minister in Chiredzi who I knew from the 'Pray for Rhodesia Campaign', told him our sad story and asked him to take Malcolm under his wing. Although I was leaving him, I did not want Malcolm to be stranded and have to sleep at the railway station.

It was so hard for me to tell Malcolm that I was finally leaving him for good and I wept as I spoke. He wept too and I held his hand but my resolve did not falter, as I really saw no future with him drinking like this. I had booked him into a home before, I had shouted and cajoled, I had pleaded and wept but nothing had worked, so I had finally come to the end. Even the police reserve reported that he was drunk most of the time at camp, so there seemed to be no hope.

Unbeknown to me a Christian mission came visiting from South Africa that weekend, after I left to go back to Fort Victoria. They visited the Methodist church in Chiredzi and according to the minister, Malcolm met them all and gave his heart to the Lord, before he went to Harare to try and find another job.

It was a sad time for all of us as we truly loved Malcolm very much. He was such a warm, loving person when he was sober. He found a job on Sanyati Estates north of Gwelo and as long as he was not drinking I decided to give it another try.

We had one last lovely weekend with him. It was half term at school and I loaded the children into the car and we drove through to see him.

Kenneth, now aged 13, caught a tiger fish in the Sanyati river and Douglas (11) shot his first guinea fowl which made an excellent meal. It was hot and we swam and braaied (had a barbeque) and generally had a wonderful family weekend, before the children and I had to go back to school in Fort Victoria.

It was the last time the children saw their father.

The next week he was drunk so lost his job again and I decided to go ahead and file for divorce. I had left him four times over the years because of his drinking and it was now affecting the children so badly, it was definitely time to call it quits.

We went to Gatooma to say goodbye to our friends there. I popped in to say goodbye to Malcolm at the motel where he was staying, but he was so drunk that I did not want the children to see him like that. He said he was going to Harare to find a job.

Later that same day, I was phoned by Sanyati Estates to say that Malcolm had had a car accident on his way to Harare, and he was not expected to live.

We immediately left to stay with friends, John and Jill Morris, who had moved from Gatooma to Harare. They took us in, and gave us such loving support at this time.

Malcolm had had the car accident on a straight piece of road, between Hartley and Harare, and there were no other cars involved. The amazing thing is that there was a policeman travelling right behind him, who saw it all. Malcolm was speeding and suddenly veered off the road and went into the bush and into a tree.

The policeman had a drip in his car, which was in itself a miracle, and he was able to put up the drip before the ambulance arrived. The doctor said he would never have survived to get to hospital, if this had not been done, as his injuries were so severe.

I drove straight to Harare as soon as I heard the news, and although I first had to drop the children off at our friends, I was still at the hospital as Malcolm was brought in. When I saw him wheeled in, I felt strangely removed from him as if he was not my husband anymore, because this time I was determined to go through with the divorce.

As the children were not allowed in the intensive care unit and, therefore, could not see their father, I put them on a plane for Cape Town the following day, to stay with my parents. I felt I should stay as long as Malcolm was alive.

I knew all the ministers in Harare because of the 'Pray for Rhodesia Campaign' and as Malcolm was a Presbyterian, I called the Presbyterian Minister, George Hamilton. Such a nice man, warm and caring, and he came at once.

Malcolm had broken all his ribs and had one punctured lung. His right leg was so badly broken that the doctors said that if he survived, it would always be shorter than the other. He had severe concussion but was conscious when George and I saw him in the intensive care unit.

Malcolm had never been keen on coming to church with me but the minister in Chiredzi believed his recent conversion at the mission was genuine. George asked him now if he had given his heart to the Lord Jesus, and if Jesus was his Lord, and he nodded his head slightly. George prayed for him and then the nurse shooed us out. That night George Hamilton had a heart attack and landed in hospital himself.

I called in the Anglican minister, as I was an Anglican. Father Joe came to see Malcolm but he was now in a coma, and there was no response. Joe prayed for him and left, phoning me that night to say he would go and see Malcolm again, but that he was feeling ill and probably wouldn't make it next day. The following day I phoned to find out how he was, and heard that Father Joe had pneumonia and was confined to bed for at least two weeks.

I was perplexed. Now who did I call in to pray for Malcolm? I remembered how alone and abandoned I had felt in hospital when I asked for a minister and no one came. I really felt I needed to get someone.

I remembered Gary Strong, a charismatic Methodist Minister. My friend Jill and I had gone to a couple of his evening meetings and I felt he would be good for Malcolm. I phoned him and was astounded to hear him say, after a short silence on the line.
"Helen, the Lord has told me not to come and pray for Malcolm."
I burst into tears and pleaded with him but he remained adamant.
"I am sorry, but I cannot do what the Lord tells me not to do." He said.

I had found a job and every evening I went to see Malcolm but it was a duty visit as I had already cut myself off from him mentally and emotionally. He came out of the coma and slipped back again, and the doctor told me that the next coma would probably be the end.

Who could I get to come and pray for Malcolm? I thought of Alistair Geddes who had a large charismatic church and I phoned him.
"Yes, certainly, I will come and see your husband but I am organizing a big conference with Pastor Alexander Bell from Scotland so I am very, very busy but I will come, I promise."

Well I waited and waited and no one came. I phoned him again and he said he would come that very afternoon but he did not come.

I walked into the intensive care ward that evening and stood at the door. The sister on duty looked straight through me, as if she did not see me, and then she just walked out of the room. This was the first time I had ever been left quite alone with Malcolm. There was no movement from the bed and the respirator made soft swooshing noises as it worked, keeping him alive. The drips and other machines around his bed were intimidating.

I took one step forward into the room and God spoke to me in my heart.
"You pray for him."
"Oh, I can't Lord. I am divorcing him and he will soon not be my husband."
"You pray for him."
"No, Lord, really I don't know what to say."
"You pray for him."
With every step, the voice became more insistent until I was at the foot of Malcolm's bed and I knew that I had to do it.
"Alright Lord, I will pray for him."

I went up to Malcolm and took his hand.
"Lord God" I started not knowing what to say.
Immediately I felt the presence of the Lord around us. Jesus was standing on the other side of the bed facing me and His Spirit enveloped us all around. I could almost see Him, He was so real. There was no light or outward manifestation but I knew without a shadow of doubt that God was there with us. I could feel a powerful, loving presence.

All the anger and distress left my heart and I felt a tremendous peace. I know Malcolm felt it too and I saw his body relax and the tears slip under his closed eyelids, as I started to pray. My love for him welled up again, poured out towards him and I felt his love for me joining in a total reconciliation. There was warmth and love between us, and the words came easily as I prayed and talked to him. When I told him about the children and how they sent their love and were praying for him, the tears rolled faster. He really loved his children.

I stayed there holding his hand, praying and talking, until the tears stopped and I could see complete rest come into him. I kissed him gently on the forehead and left. I felt at peace at last.

Malcolm died a few hours later after being in intensive care for six weeks.

I learned later from a friend, Edna Holderness, who was at Pastor Bell's crusade, that Alistair Geddes could not attend any of the meetings at all. He had had a motor bike accident while on his way to see someone in hospital!

Gary Strong phoned me to apologize for refusing to come and pray for Malcolm but he was right and obedient to the Lord as I told him when I told him the story.

It is mind blowing to think God went to so much trouble to ensure that I pray for my husband, so that there would be complete restoration between us. I now know that Malcolm has gone to be with the Lord.

After the funeral I went to Cape Town to be with my parents and my children. For about three years I still felt guilty about Malcolm, as I knew he had had the accident because he was drunk and he was drinking more because I had finally decided to divorce him. However at last I accepted that I was forgiven, and my guilt was washed away. It was Psalm 103 that spoke to me again. God told me He had forgiven all my sins and removed all my iniquity from me.

Malcolm was 43 years old when he died and the children were 13, 11 and 9. Kenneth, the eldest, has battled the most without his father, but all my children have given their hearts to the Lord, so they have a Heavenly Father to care for them.

One day we will all see Malcolm again.

Joy and her husband, Clyde, went to visit the farm in the Happy Valley before they immigrated to Australia, and Malcolm's ashes were scattered on a hill, amongst the flame lilies, overlooking the green fields of the valley. God undertook for Malcolm's life and his salvation.

I went to Cape Town to start a new life. I took very little with me as I sold everything I could, to raise a bit of capital to take with me. I arrived in Cape Town after a long trip, first by train to Johannesburg, and then by plane.

I was exhausted, mentally, spiritually and physically.

Chapter Eight

A Miracle Child

We moved to Cape Town and stayed with my parents who had a three bed roomed house overlooking the river and vlei, only a couple of blocks from the sea, in Muizenberg on the False Bay Coast. It is a beautiful area dominated by the towering Muiz Mountain with Table Mountain on the northern horizon. I used what little capital I had brought out of Zimbabwe, to build another garage onto Mom's home and turn the existing garage into two bedrooms and a bathroom for the boys.

My parents were marvellous the way they took us in, and the children went to the local schools which were within walking distance. We got on well as a family but we all had to learn housework as there was not the full time domestic help that we were accustomed to in Zimbabwe.

We experienced a wonderful new freedom, far from the war, although the first time I heard the guns going off at the Simonstown Naval Base, I actually dropped to the ground, which was the standard practice when we heard gunfire in Zimbabwe. It was such a relief not to be obliged to carry guns and be constantly on the alert for ambushes and attacks.

My first responsibility in Cape Town was to find work. I was not trained for anything as I had married at 19 and left university after one year. Now I had nothing and had three children to support. I discovered that I had a flair for sales so made that my career. I did a Marketing Management Diploma at the Cape Technical College and became a sales manager with an insurance company.

This phase of our new life in South Africa was sadly disrupted by my parents' divorce. This was a great shock to me and very painful and I began to understand what my children must have suffered as a result of the breakdown of my marriage with their father, especially as my filing for divorce had preceded Malcolm's fatal accident. We all had to heal from the past.

Now started the part of my life that I am definitely not proud of. We continued staying with my mother and I became what we call in South Africa "a joller". I joined a club, 'Parents without Partners', and went to every party I could find, dancing till all hours. This became my form of exercise to keep trim and fit. I was 35 and attractive, with lots of boyfriends and I did the rounds from one to the other. I was sowing my wild oats and I became like an irresponsible teenager again, going out as often as I could, leaving the children with my mother. Kenneth still loves to tell the story of how his friends thought I was his sister.

I was burning the candle at both ends, and in the middle, so it was not surprising that I landed up in Groote Schuur Hospital with another attack of MS. I was definitely not walking as I should before the Lord. In fact God had been very patient and understanding with me, allowing me to recover from Malcolm's death in this unorthodox manner, but my lifestyle invited the enemy to come in and make me ill again.

This was not a very severe attack but it was a big wake up call and I realized that if I did not get my life right, I would not recover from MS and I would land up where I did not want to be… paralyzed. I started going to church again and found a boy friend who would come with me. I got better and I got close to the Lord again.

My relationship with Dick was stormy and steamy but because he came to church, I thought he was the right one. We got engaged and I broke it off three times but eventually we set a wedding date.

In January 1980 there was a Christian Charismatic Conference in Johannesburg and I arranged to go with a group from our Charismatic Anglican church. We were all booked in various hotels and the conference was being held at the old show grounds in Milner Park. It was at this conference that I was finally healed of the guilt I felt about Malcolm's death. Reinhardt Bonke prayed for me and God touched me with forgiveness that I could feel deep in my being.

It was terribly hot at the conference. There were about 8000 people there and not enough water readily available for so many to drink between lectures, and I developed cystitis, a bladder infection, to which I was prone.

I couldn't afford to go to a doctor or a chemist, and anyway I did not want to miss any lectures, so I went to the early prayer meeting at our hotel and asked them to pray for me. "I know God heals because He has healed me of Multiple Sclerosis. Please, would you pray for me now so that this cystitis goes away?" I asked them.

They prayed for me and, sure enough, the bladder infection disappeared immediately and I had no more problems at all.

However I developed an enormous bruise on my stomach.

When I was first diagnosed with MS, the doctors decided that I must not have any more children, and as I had three beautiful children anyway, I agreed to have my tubes cut and tied. The doctors in Gatooma believed in doing a thorough job and, when I woke up from the anaesthetic, I discovered I had a long scar similar to a hysterectomy cut. This bruise, I had now, was right over the scar and it looked as if someone had punched me.

I pressed the bruise but it was not painful at all. It was just there, a great big black and blue bruise. I forgot about it during the day and enjoyed the conference. It was only as I dressed and undressed that I saw and wondered what it was. When I got back to Cape Town, I decided to have it checked out and went to the doctor. He examined me, pressed my tummy but could find nothing wrong.

Dick and I got married, with my children walking me into the church and giving me away. It was a lovely wedding with all our work colleagues and the church congregation bringing plates of eats. My Dad provided the champagne and my stepmother the flowers for the tables and my mother was sweet and gentle towards them both. We went to Franschhoek on honeymoon and I was immediately pregnant.

What I think happened at the conference, is that the Lord said, "Sure I will heal your cystitis but while I am about it, I will just heal everything in that area as well, so you can have another child". He might even have allowed the cystitis, so I would go for prayer and He could heal me. Whatever was on God's mind, I know He did it.

Because my tubes had been cut and tied, God had to cut and rejoin them so there was bleeding and a bruise, but because God did the operation, there was no pain or any discomfort. God gave me the bruise to show that He had done the work. Even the gynaecologist said it was a miracle. After tubes are cut and tied as mine were, the chances are about four hundred thousand to one that a woman will conceive.

God gave us a miracle child and when I was 40 years old, Ramsay was born, 13 years younger than my daughter Joy.

Joy became Ramsay's surrogate mother, wheeling him around Muizenberg in his push chair where ever she went. Kenneth was 17 and became head boy of his school and leader of the Christian Youth group so we were all very proud of him. Douglas, with a lovely nature, was a sociable guy, proving to be a good sportsman as well as very bright at school. Both boys were keen surfers and would even go down to surf before school if the waves were good. They were happy, well adjusted children, I thought, despite what they had been through. I was proud of their good manners, good character and open friendly natures.

The marriage was not a success, however, and I soon found out that Dick was not only a heavy social drinker, which I knew before we got married, and was the reason I had broken the engagement so many times, but he was also a womanizer. Although he had come to church with me and professed Christianity, he was not really a Christian at all and his life style was anything but Christian. What a fool I had been but I had my miracle Ramsay and I had made my bed and must lie on it.

Life in our household became very difficult. We had a new marriage, a new baby, 3 teenagers in the house and my mother. Dick was transferred to Johannesburg and we sold the house in Muizenberg and moved away from our friends and church, and the children had to start in new schools. My mother came with us because I did not want to leave her on her own in Cape Town. Kenneth went to the army and then the Navy, and my mother kept out of the way as much as possible, but it was still a very crowded house. I was working for a direct marketing health company but finances were very tight as Dick was out every night and did not contribute much to the household expenses.

Johannesburg was totally different from Cape Town. There were advantages like a wonderful climate where gardens grow beautifully, but it was noisy and busy and we all missed the sea and the mountains and lovely scenery in the Cape. I went to church and home group regularly, but there was no time for me to spend with God in my Airplane and my peace and joy in the Lord were dissipating.

My mother always seemed well and cheerful, despite her arthritis, and she loved doing the gardening and spoiling Ramsay with special titbits she kept in her room. We didn't have time for sitting and chatting and it seemed that we moved past each other, as we got on with our busy lives. So Mom, sensibly, made her own life and joined the Baptist Church, where she was very active and had many friends. Her independence was curtailed, however, when she was 80 and we had to stop her driving because she tended to bump into other cars when trying to park ("Just a little bump" she said.), and there were complaints from people at the shopping centre.

One day when I got back from work, my mother was missing. Nobody knew where she was and I walked and drove around the neighbourhood for hours looking for her. At last I called at a filling station close by and discovered that she had walked there, and asked them to take her to hospital because she was feeling ill, and she didn't want to call me from work.

I immediately drove to the hospital, only to discover that they had put her to lie down in a ward and forgotten all about her. By the time I got there, the doctors had all gone off duty and no one had attended to her.

She was vomiting blood and in great pain so I took her straight to the Johannesburg General Hospital. She was seen immediately and after extensive tests and x-rays, they said her gall bladder had burst and she must have an emergency operation. Douglas and Joy were with me but had to go home and I stayed alone by my mother's side.

Although it was only a couple of hours before she was wheeled into theatre, it was time enough for me to share my love and thanks to her, for my happy childhood and the knowledge and faith in God she had given me. I, truly, could never have got through my life without it, and I got it all from her. The most precious gift a parent can ever give a child. She died the next day, never recovering consciousness after the operation.

Mom's funeral was like a revival meeting. All her friends from church were there and the neighbours, who came out of respect, had a glimpse of a true Christian's send off to heaven. We were all happy for her as we knew where she was. Our sense of loss and sorrow was over shadowed by the joy of celebrating a long and faithful life in the service of her Saviour and Lord. All her family came to the funeral and the reunion was itself a joy and a comfort. Even my Dad came up to the funeral.

Dick retreated to the caravan with a six pack of beers during the remembrance party, and shortly afterwards I found out about his latest girl friend (one of many) and I put my foot down.
"Choose either me or her." I said.
He moved in with her and I filed for divorce.

Costa Mitchell, who was the marketing manager of the nutrition company where I worked, was a great help to me during this period. You can imagine the stress of both the death of my mother and the divorce all at once. Of course I landed in hospital again with an MS attack. It might sound as if I went from one attack to another but, in between times, I was perfectly well and able to live a full active life.

This was a bad attack, however, and I couldn't walk or drive and lost sensation in all my limbs. I phoned Professor Aimes in Cape Town and she said I must go to Johannesburg General Hospital to the neurology department and speak to Professor Reef. Once again I had all the tests including an MRI scan which showed lots of little scabs on my brain, typical of MS.

They put me onto cortisone, immuran, and all the tablets that prevent side effects and this time they tried the hyperbaric chamber.

The hyperbaric chamber is like a glass coffin in which oxygen is pumped at very high pressure. It is quite frightening, and after they took me into the room to explain the procedure, I actually wrote out my will! But while lying there (like Snow White), I prayed for the Lord to keep me safe, and the doctors told me, that I was the first one ever to fall asleep during the treatment.

I just imagined myself lying on a cloud with God's everlasting arms holding me up. Before I knew it, I was fast asleep. I also learnt not to be stressed by the prodding, poking and knee banging, the fluffy feathers and pricking needles of the examinations. I rested in the Lord through it all and this I know is the secret God taught me; but...

Depression is one of the symptoms of this illness as all MS sufferers will tell you. It is a physiological depression because your brain is attacked and sick. I had always been protected from it because of my bubbling joy in the Lord, but this time, as a result of the trauma I had just gone through, the depression hit me.

My mother was gone, my husband had gone off with another woman and I was alone with Ramsay, now a six year old. Ken was in the navy and Doug and Joy were working and studying at university and lived full independent lives.

I felt abandoned, but at the same time enclosed in a small, black steel box, dark and cold as night. I was discharged from hospital but was still ill and in bed at home.

I prayed and came before the Lord, in agony of soul, for Him somehow to help me out of this terrible blackness. I felt I had come to the end, my life was useless and I had had enough. I couldn't go on anymore. I wasn't any use to anyone and I just wanted to die.

Chapter 9

Radio Pulpit

I hadn't heard the voice of the Lord for a long time now. I had been too wrapped up in my life, work, and problems to spend the quality time I needed with Him. I had never stopped going to church, and people at work knew I was a Christian, as I never ceased to witness, but I had not spent enough real communication time with Him. I had forgotten about God's constant presence and had climbed out of my Airplane.

Now as I called out to Him in my deep depression I heard His voice again.

"Pick up your Bible." He said

I picked up my Bible and it fell open to Luke chapter 5. There I read the story of Jesus telling his disciples to cast their nets out into the lake again, even if they had caught nothing all night. They did so and caught so many fish, that their nets were breaking, and they filled two boats until they were almost sinking.

I asked God what this meant for me and I got the answer that I must change my job and go out to catch fish (Evangelism? Work for Him?)
"Where do you want me to work, Lord?" I asked
I had no idea where He wanted me to go. I had my car radio permanently tuned on Radio Pulpit so I could get the Word of God whenever I was in the car, and I now heard God's voice saying, "Radio Pulpit."

I was excited and my depression vanished. God said I must go and work for Radio Pulpit! I was only too happy to be obedient.

I didn't even know where the head office of Radio Pulpit was, and I certainly didn't know what the phone number was, but I am not one to allow the grass to grow under my feet when I have a message from the Lord. I was so excited and happy. I hadn't heard Him for so long and it was wonderful hearing His voice talking to me again.

I phoned directory enquiries and got Radio Pulpit's phone number.

The girl who answered the phone there must have thought I was crazy, as I was short and to the point.
I gave my name and said, "The Lord has told me that I must come and work for Radio Pulpit."
They must get a lot of crack pot phone calls like that because her only comment was.

"But you're English."

"Sure, I'm English. What has that got to do with it? The Lord has told me to come and work for you."

"We only have Afrikaans people working here."

"You have English on the radio. Why can't you have English people working for you?"

There was silence and then she asked "What do you do now?

"I am in sales. I am a sales manager."

"Oh well, let me put you through to the sales department." She was obviously pleased to pass this one on.

They put me through to Mr Piet van Jaarsveld and he was just as off putting.

"We do have sales people but they are only Afrikaans."

I repeated, "God has told me to come and work for you."

"Well…. you can go for an interview. If you live in Johannesburg you will fall under Dominee Kosie Loots and you will have to go through to Germiston to see him and if he thinks you are suitable then you come for an interview with me."

He gave me Dominee Kosie's phone number, I thanked him and said goodbye. Germiston was quite a way and I was still too ill to drive.

I was shaking and depressed all over again. I must have heard the Lord wrongly. They obviously didn't want me. I was back to square one, back in my cold black depression. Then I heard the Lord again, "Pick up your bible."

I lay back on the pillows exhausted. Was this all worth it? I couldn't even hear the Lord properly anymore.

Half heartedly, I did what I was instructed and picked up my bible. It fell open to John chapter 21 and the words jumped out bold before my eyes; the similar story of Jesus telling his disciples to cast their nets on the other side of the boat and he would give them many fish.

I sat bolt upright in bed. This was no mistake. This was definitely the Lord telling me again. He did want me to go and work for Radio Pulpit.
"OK, Lord, thank you. You have shown me, now You must just show them as well. Thank you Lord."

When I was well enough, I went from interview to interview and filled out reams of application forms all in Afrikaans. I got on well with Dominee Kosie and Oom Piet van Jaarsveld but I could see that they were most perplexed about the idea of having an English PRO, which is what they called their sales people. My Afrikaans was poor but their English was better and we managed to communicate quite well, so I left it all to the Lord. His will be done.

I recovered my health and sold my mother's grand piano to keep food on the table. Three months later they phoned me to say that I had been accepted.

My job at Radio Pulpit was to find sponsors for the programs. We could either do this in the form of debit orders from individuals on a monthly basis, or go to companies who would sponsor different programs on an annual basis. I preferred the companies as the amount was obviously larger, and I made my target more easily. The debit orders were given mostly by the Afrikaans community and it was after-hours work, so I didn't do too well there.

However if I went to prayer groups meeting in the work place, I could give out debit order forms, and leave people to pray about it and post their forms. If my code was on the form I still got credited with the income. This is how my ministry in the prayer groups started. There were a lot of prayer groups in Johannesburg and I phoned up big companies to find them, and was also referred by prayer groups I had already seen.

I was also involved in a group of ladies who went into a suburb of Soweto, where the black people lived. We gave out soup and food from a small church, and then walked around praying for the people. We would go house to house, and it was really exciting seeing so many give their hearts to the Lord and become born again. There were miracles of healing too. One little boy, who had an enormous swelling on his head, was completely healed, and the swelling went down immediately after Lorna, our leader, laid hands on him and we all prayed. How we rejoiced and praised the Lord.

It was here that I met my prayer partner, June Gray.
June had a vision for me at one of our prayer meetings in Soweto. She said she saw a house on a hill with light shining out of the windows lighting the dark around. She said the Lord had given her the interpretation that the house was me, built on the rock of Christ and shining His light to the people around me, who were in the darkness. I was so thrilled. This confirmed God's word to me that I was in the right place with Radio Pulpit.

I was so grateful for this encouragement from the Lord and thereafter June and I would pray together at my home before I addressed a prayer group, and we would go together in her car, as my old car was always giving trouble. Then she would sit in the back of the room and pray while I was talking and we would pray together for people who wanted prayer.

I started by telling people about Radio Pulpit, and how many letters we got from people who were helped and came to the Lord, through this ministry. Then I would pass out the debit order forms and ask people to support Radio Pulpit on a monthly basis.

Afterwards I would give them my testimony of healing and what God had done for me. Many people came forward for prayer for healing and God healed there too. One lady with a back problem, who needed to have an operation, was healed and never had to have the operation at all. Another with gall bladder problems and a man with kidney stones were among those, I can remember, who were totally healed. We did not hear about the healings in all the prayer groups, but when we went back, we got word that God had healed there as well.

I spoke about what God had taught me about abiding in the vine and God's Airplane, and what He had taught me about prayer. The presence of the Lord was always so strong and God gave words of prophesy through us as well. It was a wonderful time of walking with the Lord. I would never have had the courage to do it on my own but Jesus sent people out two by two, and with constant back up of prayer from June, I knew that God was always with us. In His power I had the courage to talk and teach, and together we could pray for people.

I never had so much as a twinge of MS during this time.

There was one amazing God-incidence to show me the power of prayer. I was at home one evening when the phone rang quite late and a lady asked to speak to Joy. I explained that Joy was out and she said her name was Belinda and she knew Joy from work, and could I, please, ask Joy to phone her when she came home. She sounded so distressed and there was obviously something very wrong so I asked if I could help her.

She went on to explain that she lived on a small holding in Roodepoort (the other side of Johannesburg), She was alone and there were people trying to break into her house. She had phoned the police but no on had come and she was terrified. I asked her if I could pray for her and she said "Yes. Please"
The Lord said to me "The blood of Jesus" but I prayed that the protection of Jesus would be over her.
She cried, "They are coming closer. I can hear them at the window."
I prayed that the presence and the peace of Jesus be with her.
She shouted, panic stricken, "They are coming. They have broken the window."
At last I prayed that the blood of Jesus would cover her and her home and there was immediate peace in her. I could feel it over the telephone.

"They are going. They have gone. Thank you. Thank you Lord."

It was the blood of Jesus which was effective.

A few minutes later she said, "The police have just arrived. Oh thank you. Oh thank you Lord"

My daughter, Joy did not know anyone by her name or anyone at all living in Roodepoort. How did she get our number?

There were times of protection for me as well. Once when I was addressing a prayer group at the library in central Johannesburg, June was away, and there was a riot outside the building. The prayer group leader begged me to stay, as he said it was not safe for me to leave. I felt the Lord saying He would protect me, and after they prayed for me I left. The front door was locked against the rioters, and the security guard really did not want to let me out, but I was quite peaceful and unafraid. I walked into that maelstrom of seething, angry black humanity saying aloud with every step.

"Thank you Jesus, Praise you Jesus, Bless you Jesus."

The people just parted for me and I had a clear pathway to the garage where I had parked my car.

In the parking garage, I asked the attendant if he knew Jesus and we had a long conversation. He asked me why the devil was always depicted as black. Did that mean that they, as black men were associated with the devil? I prayed and God gave me the words. I explained that it had nothing to do with the colour of a man's skin as God looks upon the heart. God is goodness and light and in Him there is no evil or darkness so God judged people according to the goodness (light) or evil (darkness) of their hearts.

The devil was all evil so his heart was black with evil and he was depicted as black, but he could masquerade as an angel of light if he wanted to. There were white people and all colour people who had black evil hearts, and there were many black people who had given their hearts to Jesus and therefore their hearts were white with God's righteousness. I explained that Jesus had come to die for all people, whatever the colour of their skin, and that he loved all humankind and wanted them all to be saved from sin, and come to the knowledge of the loving Father God, and have a personal relationship with Him.

This was the time of the struggle of the black people in South Africa and this man did not want me to pray for him but he took in everything that I said, and I do hope that sometime that seed came to harvest. I am sure he was the reason God wanted me to brave the riots to get back to my car.

We lived in 9th Road, Kew, very close to Alexandra Township and we often heard guns going off in the township. One day when I was taking my char home with a bag of oranges and food for her family, I was accosted, my handbag stolen and the thieves tried to get my car keys from me. I was angry but not afraid and tried to throw my keys to the char but she was too terrified and ran away as fast as she could. One man picked up my keys but I followed him and tried to get them back from him.

I beat him on the chest in frustration when he held them over his head. I cried out that I was a Christian and was trying to help his people but when I saw the look in his eyes, I knew I was in danger. I cried out to God to help me. Just then a white car came down the normally deserted road and the thieves ran away with my bag and keys. I stayed beside my car and an army vehicle came and parked with me until I could get a locksmith to change the locks.

People said I was crazy to fight back and I should have just let them take my car, but God protected me and I and my car were unharmed.

I was not afraid at the time but reaction set in and for a couple of months I looked over my shoulder wherever I went. However I knew that God had kept me safe and He was with me in danger.

I was also tricked out of my bank card at the ATM and R2000 was stolen out of my account but God showed me that I had no reason to be afraid as long as I lived in the shadow of His wings.

I could ill afford any loss of money, as I was now a single mom, supporting my children with no maintenance from my ex husband, but God told me He would provide for me. Kenneth was now in the navy, Douglas was doing his articles and studying to be an accountant, and Joy was at university and waitressing part time to help pay her way.

I made a list of all my debts and needs and prayed over it asking God specifically to provide. The total came to

R7000, double what I earned in a month, so I had no way of getting this money apart from a miracle of God.

We had a sauna in the back garden next to the swimming pool but we never used it. A couple of weeks later the sauna burnt down. We never found out what caused the fire. There was a tremendous amount of smoke and flames roared into the air and threatened to engulf the house as well. Fire engines came roaring but couldn't get into the back garden, and eventually had to park in the street and run their hoses over the garden gate. The fire was put out just in time before the roof of the house caught alight.

The insurance on the sauna came to exactly R7000 and God supplied all my financial need as I had asked.

Chapter 10

Learning to Forgive

My personal life though, was at an all time low. I felt so guilty being a Christian, working for Radio Pulpit and being divorced. God had given us a miracle child so surely He wouldn't let the marriage disintegrate like this. Perhaps we could still make it work. Dick and I started talking and Douglas and Joy left home in protest. They had supported me during my divorce and didn't want to see me getting back with Dick again.

Dick moved out from his girlfriend and took a garden cottage and Ramsay and I went to visit him and we spent a couple of Sundays with him. Reconciliation seemed the right thing and I married him for the second time 18months after the divorce. I sold the house in Kew and bought another smaller one in Fishers Hill, Germiston, thinking that a different environment would help with a fresh start.

Ramsay and I were the only two living at home now, so Dick could no longer blame the rest of the family for his constant absences from home. However things were as bad as ever and when I went to pick Ramsay up from school I used to see his car parked outside the pub at lunch time. He wasn't even putting in a full day's work and it was the same old story. I popped in there to see one day and he was even flirting with other women again.

I made the decision to divorce him again after only three years of the second marriage when Ramsay was 10 years old. Ramsay supported my decision as he was old enough now to know what was going on. We took in a series of boarders to help pay the bills and we made a new life.

However, I battled to get free from Dick emotionally and during counselling I learned about the soul ties which are formed when there are sexual bonds. I was prayed for, to have these soul ties broken, but I didn't have much relief. I still found myself thinking of him far too much and wanting to contact him, although he now lived with another girlfriend who later became his next wife.

The stress of a second divorce brought on another MS attack and I was admitted to hospital again. Dick came to see me, bringing flowers, magazines and chocolates and I was so low that I was tempted to see him again. Would I never get free of this man who was so wrong for me and brought me nothing but unhappiness?

When I was out of hospital, I sat up in bed one night and asked God to help me.

"Please, Lord, help me get free from this relationship. Show me the reason I am still tied to him."

"You can't get free because you have not forgiven him for what he has done to you. You are bound by memories and un-forgiveness." God said.

"But, Lord. I thought I had forgiven that is why I remarried him. Nevertheless if that is what You say, please Lord, will You teach me how to forgive properly." I asked.

At once, God started playing videos in my mind of my life together with Dick from the very beginning, showing me things that I thought I had forgotten. With each scene there was a heavy blackness in my heart, as God took me through every detail and told me to forgive.

"I forgive you, Dick, for what you did on that occasion. and how you hurt me." As I said it, the blackness lifted slightly.

"Forgive me, Lord, for my anger against him." The burden lifted a little more.

"I forgive myself for my reactions and my anger even if I buried it and said nothing." The heaviness lifted a little bit more and I knew I was on the right track.

"I forgive all the other persons involved and the cause of the incident."

The Lord showed me that I must even forgive the inanimate causes of an incident, for example alcohol, as well as the other woman or drinking mates that were involved. Anything that caused anger or anguish while reliving the experience in the vision, had to be forgiven. As I did this, the blackness lifted more but it was still there and I did not know what else to do.

"I have forgiven, Lord, what more must I do?" I asked.

"Remember what I said on the cross. Father, forgive them for they know not what they do."

"But, Lord, he did know what he was doing, I had already spoken to him. He knew that it was wrong and that he was causing me pain by his actions." I said.

"So did the people who condemned me to death and nailed me the cross." The Lord replied. "Dick did not understand the depth of hurt and damage to you, so he did not know in full what he was doing. If you cannot ask Me to forgive him you are in essence saying, 'Lord I forgive him but You get him for what he did.' That is not **My** kind of forgiveness. I want you to forgive completely in the same way as I give complete forgiveness to you through the cross. That will set you free."

"Oh, Lord, I am sorry. I see it now." I said and prayed. "Father please will You forgive him because he did not know what he was doing."

Immediately the heaviness lifted and the dark burden had gone.

I had to go through every memory video that the Lord brought to me. It took me a whole night, the next day and half of the second night before I was through. Then I slept like a baby and next morning woke up totally refreshed and free.

The Lord showed me in this way that we will never be free of our past hurts, including childhood damage, unless we completely forgive the people and situations that have hurt us. We must ask God to forgive them as well. I believe this is what Jesus meant when he said "Pray for those who despitefully use you." And "If you do not forgive you will not be forgiven". We cannot be healed physically, emotionally or spiritually if we do not forgive completely.

This is what was preventing the final part of my healing. With forgiveness there is a freedom from the past, freedom from soul ties and hurts; freedom from anger, bitterness and resentment, however deeply buried. This is what causes our separation from God and is, in many cases, the cause of our sickness and diseases.

I have taught this in motivational courses to people with childhood trauma and it is amazing how it has freed them, when they follow this pattern. I just praise God for this inner healing and His grace in showing it to me.

Psychiatrists tell us we must work through our past, but reliving it does not heal, it only entrenches the scars unless we forgive every person who has hurt us. Forgiving God's way is the only way to be healed and get free from the pain of the past. Forgiveness and abiding in Christ are the paths to healing.

I was asked on many occasions to go and see people who were suffering from MS. I would go if the patient herself/ himself phoned me. Then I knew they were really interested in how I was healed. Before I made that rule I went to see people who were wallowing in self pity who did not want to hear what I was saying. They listened but did not hear and would not do what I had done. It was too much effort for them.

God does intervene miraculously in some people's lives for healing and protection, before they are born again, but I discovered that the first thing for my kind of healing is to really believe in Jesus Christ and be born again. Hebrews 11:6 says "Without faith it is impossible to please God, for whoever would draw near to God, must believe that He exists and that He rewards those who seek Him". To meet Jesus in a personal way is the beginning of faith.

Our natural sin and prideful natures are separating us from God. It is only through the realization of the complete forgiveness of God through what Jesus did for us, that we can truly come to God. We cannot be healed by Him if we do not come to Him. We have to have an appointment with our Doctor and see and speak to Him face to face.

The second thing is that we must really want to get well. Unfortunately I met some people who actually enjoyed their helplessness and enjoyed being waited on hand and foot. Of course, they did not see this, as their self pity closed their eyes and ears, and refused to let them see what was in their hearts.

Their illness consumed them spiritually as well as physically, and they could not see the greatness of God and His love above the physical manifestations of MS. They kept their eyes on themselves and the illness, rather than on God. We need to look beyond ourselves, our illness and symptoms if we want to be healed. This is difficult because the illness is there to see and feel, whereas God is unseen. We have to get to know God, His reality and His Love before we can see Him above our suffering.

We have to know in heart and mind that God is good, that He loves us and doesn't want His children sick and suffering. He wants us well and happy with abundant life.

I met one girl with MS who was consumed by anger against her husband who would not pander to her every whim and come running at her beck and call. She thought this was her right because of her illness. I have mentioned the anger and volatility of one's emotions in this illness, and temper, selfishness and self pity have to be fought.

How terrible to live with a selfish person who makes everyone miserable; How much more, a sick demanding person who appears to blame the world and everyone in it, constantly demanding the retribution of slavish attention. That person has the wrong attitude.

I also met people who thought it was just too much trouble and effort to study God's word and let it sink into their subconscious. The Bible calls it renewing our minds and if we want healing, we must do it. I was just so blessed because God put His love and faith in me and it was an absolute delight to sit with Him and read His word. We must ask God for this gift of faith and joy to study His word and pray for the Holy Spirit to enlighten us.

Some of the people I counselled would read and study half-heartedly for a week or so and then go back to reading escapist novels that took their mind off their problems but certainly did not solve their problems like God does.

I lent people books (and lost many) but they did not read them or didn't finish reading them. It was very puzzling to me because this for me was the food and drink that had made me well. I couldn't understand why some people would not put in the effort to read and study the word for their own healing. Anyway it was their choice. At first I really got upset and tried my best to motivate them, until I realized some people just wouldn't do it.

Then there were the people who were already defeated and saw no hope for healing even after seeing me and hearing my story. They could not believe it when I told them I had not been able to walk at all for two years and that it took another 3 years before I got back on the tennis court to knock a few balls. They couldn't relate to my present good health and some, I think, even thought I was fabricating the whole thing. They did not want to believe. It is so sad.

Some people were angry with God and blamed Him for their illness. This was very difficult to counsel because the more I said that God does not bring sickness and that Satan does, the more they told me that if He was an Almighty God He was responsible for everything. I told them that God had allowed Satan to bring the disease, in the same way He had allowed Satan to put boils on Job, but they still blamed God. They could not see, or did not want to see, that until they were covered by the blood of Jesus when they were born again, Satan had a legal right to get at them because man had turned his back on God.

I explained that in some cases our reaction to circumstances, allowing stress, worry, bitterness and un-forgiveness to consume us, had brought on the sickness. Stress is a major cause of MS and it is only as we learn to trust God and cast all our burdens on Him, and leave them there, that we are healed.

I explained that God had shown His love for us by sending His Son Jesus to take our sin, stress and sickness away, because He did not give them to us in the first place. Some people would not listen or could not hear anything above their anger at God. I got to the stage of just praying for them and asking God to show them His love and goodness. They had to believe in a loving God, a God of mercy and goodness before they could go to Him for healing.

Some people, I saw, were so immersed in their problems and misery that they could not imagine themselves well. Even when I told them to hold pictures of themselves walking and running again, they could not do it. Anyone can a put picture in his mind so I did not understand this either. Was the enemy, the devil, stopping them? He stalks around seeing who he can destroy, and he sure did destroy them.

One lovely Jewish girl refused to come to the Messiah for healing even though all of the scriptures I quoted were from the Old Testament and I never mentioned the name of Jesus. This was the condition on which she asked to see me. She was exercising and practicing walking and taking all the supplements and vitamins but refused to believe that God was a loving God who would heal. She was trying to do it herself, leaving God out of it. This is the same pride that is our greatest separation from God. She thought she could do it all herself, and didn't need God.

Some people did not even want to see me when I told them that God had healed me. They did not even want to hear.

However there were the people who listened and heard and followed a path to climb into their Jumbo Jet, Rest in the Vine and Abide in Christ. I saw their spirits lift, a glow in their eyes and an improvement in their health. I have lost touch with many of them now but it is such a privilege to bring a person hope and expectation of healing, through what Jesus has done for me.

I thank God for my experience that has drawn me so close to Him and enabled me to help others.

Chapter 11

Ministry of Healing

When June, my prayer partner, and I went to prayer meetings at businesses in Johannesburg, and I gave my testimony, we were asked to go and visit many sick people.

We were asked to pray for two very ill women; one with terminal cancer and the other with MS and breast cancer. The first lady really battled with lack of faith because her pain was so bad but I think in our weekly visits, we did help her to understand the loving heart of the Father God. I do hope so. We prayed for her constantly but the Lord took her home to be with Him. We don't know why not everyone is healed but we must always remember that this life is but a blink of an eye whereas eternity is forever and ever.

The second girl was clearly demon possessed and would go into frightening rages when we prayed for her. On one occasion when she was lying on the floor in exhaustion after one of these rages, and I was bending over her praying for her, I saw her eyes change and she actually tried to strangle me. I could do nothing but June immediately stood up and rebuked the demon and it left and our patient was quiet and peaceful in a moment. This is why God sends us out in twos.

We were puzzled by this girl because she repeatedly said she had given her heart to the Lord and she would not do it again, however much we urged her. As soon as we left, her mother said she was the same again, shouting and screaming at her all the time. There was nothing we could do without her truly repenting and wanting to get free and I think we helped her mother more than we did her. Perhaps God wanted us there just for her mother. I do not know, but we felt after a while that she was making a mockery of the Lord's grace and we stopped going. We still prayed for her and her mother, who looked after her so faithfully. I have since heard that this girl has moved to Cape Town, is healed, and has truly given her heart to the Lord and become a new creation. Thank you Lord. We planted the seed, someone else watered it and God made it grow.

With the blessing of my church, I started teaching Bible study at St Giles in Kensington. This is a home for the physically disabled and what a privilege and joy it was, to be associated with these wonderful, courageous people who were worse off, by a long shot, than I had ever been.

Jill, Bob, Dave, Mario, Celeste, Gloria, Bruce and others became an inspiration to me and I was so sad to say goodbye when we moved back to Cape Town.

The Lord taught me a wonderful lesson at St Giles. Bruce, who had MS and came to the Bible study regularly, did not say much because he battled to speak clearly. One evening he was completely lucid and we were all so pleased at his participation. It was a really happy Bible study seeing him included by everyone. We prayed for him and I laid hands on him and he had a beautiful peace and a glow I had never seen before. He died a few days later before the next Bible study and there was a sense of awe among us that God had given him this aura of happiness to show us, that he would be with Him when he went.

June and I were asked to conduct a weekend seminar on the Holy Spirit and Healing at a church in Louis Trichardt close to the Zimbabwe border. It was exciting packing up for a weekend but we were very aware of the responsibility. We prayed all the way there, a drive of about 6 hours, and just asked God to be with us and show us exactly what He wanted us to do.

I had no notes except for the teachings I had done on healing but this group of ladies specifically wanted prayer for the infilling of the Holy Spirit. I had done a Bible study on it in preparation, and June and I prayed and talked about it in the car, but I was not given a revelation and structure of what I should say, and I had to remember what Jesus said, about the Holy Spirit putting the words in my mouth. I was sorry that I was committed to do the talking and June the praying as I would have felt much better if I could have sat at the back and given her prayer support.

We were greeted with such warmth by the ladies of the church and made very comfortable in a beautiful home but I still did not know what I was going to say and I grew quite panicky as the time grew closer.
"Please, Lord, help me with what to say."
I need not to have worried. I still don't know exactly what I said but the words came and I knew it was God, not me. We prayed for people to receive the Holy Spirit and He came in power and they spoke in other tongues and went away rejoicing and glowing with the joy of the Lord.

Next day we did the healing seminar and once again the Lord moved and people were healed. It was such an honour to be instruments of God like this.

Another time I had organized for a black pastor from Radio Pulpit to speak at a meeting of housemaids at a church in a wealthy suburb of Johannesburg. I was there on time and all the lovely black ladies were on time, but after waiting for half an hour for the pastor, they were getting restive. I could not speak their language but I realized that I was going to have to talk to them and I didn't know what to say.

Once again I was panic stricken but remembered how God had spoken in Louis Trichardt so once again I said, "Lord, please, speak through me as I don't know what to say."

It was only after I had stood up, prayed and apologized for the absence of the pastor that God gave me the story of Naaman's servant girl and how she had talked to her mistress about God and been instrumental in the healing of her master.(2 Kings 5.) They were encouraged to hear that in their lowly position in a home they could still have so much influence and spread the word of God. God had once more taken over and done the talking. Thank you Lord.

One prayer group, at the Revenue Services Office in Germiston, asked me to teach them what God had taught me about healing and we had a six weeks course, where the response and the growth in the Lord amongst them, was so wonderful to see. It was an absolute blessing for us to be associated with people who loved the Lord so much and wanted to go out and help others, give them hope, faith and love from the Lord. This prayer group had wonderful healings and they brought in many others who gave their hearts to the Lord.

Some visiting Dominee, however, saw the notices of these meetings in the lift and reported me to Radio Pulpit and I was forbidden to do any more teaching. I submitted and agreed but a year later, when they told me I could no longer give my testimony, as I was giving hope and expectation to people, I was shattered. I felt I had to resign from Radio Pulpit as I must do what God told me to do, not what man told me to do.

Maybe I was acting out of hurt and pride because the truth is that God has never used me as much again, as when I was with Radio Pulpit.. I have worked with a Christian radio station here in Cape Town but without a special, dedicated prayer partner the power of the Lord has not been the same.

I believe Radio Pulpit has changed over the years and they are not so against God's spiritual gifts and His healing. I am glad as I knew many lovely Christian people there who really loved the Lord and were dedicated to His work and the furtherance of His Kingdom. May God bless them and continue working through them. Radio Pulpit does an excellent job, encouraging Christians, spreading the word of God and bringing people to the Lord.

When I was still with Radio Pulpit my father became very ill. He and my step mother, Laurine, were living in Pietermaritzburg in a granny flat with one of her daughters. We had long since mended any hurt and ill feeling over my parents divorce and I was just pleased that Dad was happy. Laurine was an excellent wife to him and I loved her as a friend.

I tried to talk to my Dad about the Lord but he had a closed mind and was into 'The Virtue of Selfishness.' Dad would get so upset when I talked to him about salvation that he almost looked as if he was going to have a heart attack. Laurine was worried about his health and I agreed to let things be. By this time, I knew that God did amazing miracles to bring His children back to Him and I asked God, that when my Dad's time came, he would be ready to call on His name. Above all I wanted my Dad to be with us in heaven and not lost in hell.

When Laurine phoned and told me my Dad was very ill and in hospital, I had an immediate urge to go down to see him. I booked on the bus leaving next morning but that night my sleep was broken with terrible dreams and visions. I saw a big black shape standing at the bottom of my Dad's bed. It was like the cowl of a monk but there was no face and just a black void under the hood. The atmosphere around this apparition was complete evil which terrified me, and I realized that it was the devil waiting for my dad to die.

I woke with a start, shivering with fear and started praying, pleading with God to keep my dad alive till he had given his heart back to Him and was saved. I lay praying in tongues and gradually drifted off to sleep again. This time I dreamed again and saw the vision of the black figure still there but I saw angels in white coming from all directions, crowding round the bed, pushing the devil away. He hung around for a while and then gradually went, floating further and further until he disappeared from my sight.

I woke again, still with an urgency to pray but the fear and desperation had gone and I had a feeling that the crisis was past. I prayed all the way down to Maritzburg and when Laurine picked me up we went straight to the hospital. Dad was propped up in bed, very pale, weak, and wan but with a smile of welcome. The sister told us that he had had to be resuscitated in the night and Dad said that he had woken up with a crowd of nurses around his bed. I knew that God had given me those visions to pray him through.

My Dad lived quite a few years after that episode. When he was 80, all the family came to a great celebration. Shortly afterwards he became friendly with a young Anglican priest and would go to the services held once a week at the Hospice. Dad died just after his 86th birthday and I know that he had made his peace with the Lord. God had taken him when he was ready to call on the name of Jesus.

Laurine is still alive and she is a wonderful friend. We correspond by fax as her hearing is not good anymore but when her time comes she will see my dad and her beloved husband again.

Chapter 12.

Final Victory

After being single for three years after the divorce, I prayed to God for a Christian husband. I had my son Ramsay, now aged 13, my friends, June, my work at Radio Pulpit and the St Giles crowd, so my life was full and rewarding but I was not a woman who could live alone and I wanted a husband and companion.

I met Bill Phillips through Leslie and Alan who were friends of mine. I invited them round to a braai (barbeque) one Sunday and they brought Bill with them. I was late because I was talking at a church and by the time I got home the fire was made and Alan was swimming in the pool. It was terribly hot and he started splashing Ramsay and me so we decided to jump in on him clothes and all. It was all great fun but Bill was very quiet and I thought he had no personality. He thought I was a "forward broad".

About six months later I met up with him again. A cellular phone company, for which I was doing Saturday morning sales training, asked me to find them a permanent Sales manager and Leslie suggested Bill.

He came round to my house at lunch time one Saturday afternoon, and Dick was there paying me a little of the maintenance he owed. He was being argumentative and critical as usual and when I was out of the room Bill told him that this was not the way to treat a woman. I knew nothing about it until later, but when I came back, Dick was gone.

When the business was out of the way, Bill and I talked. We talked and talked. It was the Rugby Curry Cup final and we watched it and talked. Ramsay was away staying with his brother Kenneth in Jeffreys Bay so we were uninterrupted. Bill had to see his sister off at the airport but he came back and we went out to dinner and talked. I discovered he had a wonderful sense of humour and a very sharp, well-informed mind.

When we got back from dinner he said," I believe you are a Christian. I have studied so many religions. Tell me about yours."
Well, I didn't need a second invitation and I started from the beginning, from the creation, fall of man, to Jesus and salvation. We sat around the dining room table and I drew diagrams and got the Bible out and looked things up. Before I knew where we were, it was 2am.

Next evening I was taking my St Giles friends to a healing service at a large church and asked Bill if he would like to come and help me load them all in the mini bus. He came and was wonderful with them, laughing and joking and making them feel special but not pitied. He handled the wheelchairs with aplomb and we arrived at the church full of laughter.

We had to sit in the front row so Bill got the best view in the 7000seater church.
"Well, what did you think?" I asked him over a cup of coffee when we got home.
"That was a well managed road show" he replied, "But still, I felt compelled to put all my money in the collection basket. I don't know why."
I left it all to the Lord.

Every evening that week, except for my St Giles evening, he came round and we talked and I answered his questions. Ramsay came home and was introduced. He was very suspicious of any man I brought home but I had brought home some weirdoes so I didn't blame him. Gradually Ramsay took to Bill.

The next Sunday I asked Bill if he would like to come to my church with me. I went to a small charismatic church in a nearby suburb, which was well organised but not a road show. John Neilson, the Pastor, was an excellent preacher and teacher and he never failed to make an altar call.

So often when you take a person to church you sit on edge, uncomfortably wondering what your guest is thinking.

This time I was totally relaxed and when it came to the altar call I closed my eyes, prayed like everyone else and was surprised when Bill put the bible on my lap and went up to the front.

His story is very interesting. He said that when he closed his eyes, he saw only black, pitch black, not the normal dark light through his eyelids. He tried to open his eyes but he couldn't. Then when John asked people to put up their hands to respond to the call, he found his arm going up involuntarily. He wanted to bring it down again but it wouldn't move and he could only open his eyes when he had to go to the front.

There were four people responding that morning and after John had led them in the sinner's prayer, he prayed for all of them individually. John was very good, in that when he prayed for people, he did not push them and sometimes did not touch them at all.

Bill was the third one to be prayed for and as John lifted his hand to pray, Bill stumbled back. If the front pew had not been there, he would have fallen. He didn't know that it was the norm to fall down when prayed for and touched by the Holy Spirit. He had never seen it before but he said he felt as if he had been hit by 2000 volts of electricity.

He came back to me dazed. "What was that?" he asked.
"You were touched by the Holy Spirit," I said
"Wow! Touched?" he said "I was zapped. I have never experienced anything like that before."

God had introduced Himself to Bill and for three days he walked around in a daze.

He was hungry for knowledge and we studied the bible together. John Neilson told him to read the Gospel of John and Proverbs to start with, we went to Wednesday evening bible study and Bill got baptized. It was a magical time and before I knew it we were in love.

I had a lovely maid called Johanna who was like a member of the family. She said in Afrikaans to me one evening, "Miesies, this is a good man. You must marry him."
I laughed and translated for Bill.
"That's a good idea," He said.
"Are you asking me to marry you?" I asked with a twinkle in my eye.
"Yes," He said and so it was agreed just like that.
Johanna had organized our engagement.

We were married a month later as neither of us saw any reason to wait. We moved back to Cape Town a year later. God gave me a husband who is kind and faithful, who was such a good father to Ramsay that he took his name and officially became his son.

As in any marriage, we have had our ups and downs but I have learnt to be a praying wife and God has been good. Bill's health is not wonderful and he has had a series of mini strokes and has to carry his angina tablets with him wherever he goes but God has been faithful and we are happy.

We are so glad to be back in Cape Town by the mountain and the sea. Muizenberg has progressed spiritually so much since we started praying for the people and places here 24 years ago. Where satanic gatherings were once commonplace, we now have a Theological college, a YWAM base, a Christian radio station, Living Hope (mission to the poor), and numerous churches.

As He has everywhere else, God has protected me here in Cape Town as well. Once when I was travelling by train a tall African man came and sat close to me on the seat and said he had a gun and I must give him my purse. He poked something into my side but once again I was not afraid and I felt the Lord saying He would protect me. I refused to give up my bag although he grabbed it and tried to pull it away from me. I stood up as the train came into my station and he stood up with me, but turned to a very frightened-looking young girl.

"Don't worry, my dear," I said to her. "I am getting off here and will call the police."

At that, the man jumped up again and came for me as I walked towards the door. He grabbed me round my body imprisoning my arms so I could not open the door.I screamed as loudly as I could and he put one hand over my mouth to muffle the sounds while still holding my arms by my side.

I prayed, "Lord help me."

The train doors opened of their own volition and, anyone knowing how heavy those doors are, would know what a miracle that was. No one touched the doors to open them;

I had my arms pinned to my sides and the man's arms were tight around me. God had saved me again. I walked off the train and the would-be robber ran off down the platform and was never seen again.

Bill lost his business in Cape Town; he lost his car and I lost my home. We started a sandwich business making sandwiches in the early hours of the morning and rushing them into Cape Town to the people working in office blocks. Bill would fetch the bread from the bakery at 4am and we worked until 10pm planning the sandwiches, making fillings and stamping labels. We were absolutely exhausted but we were making a living so we persevered.

One morning, while driving into Cape Town in the congested traffic, I was sitting praying and in my exhausted stupor I said, "Lord, I can't go on like this. You don't love me anymore."
Immediately His voice resounded in my heart, "Didn't I die for you?"
The words hit me in the solar plexus and I felt so ashamed. "Yes, Lord. I am sorry. Yes, you did die for me and I am so grateful, Lord, and I love you."
I have never doubted His love since, however hard times have been.

It was during this time of extreme financial hardship that God enabled me to forgive Dick in one final area, the area of finances.

When Bill lost his business, we were so poor that I renewed my efforts to get maintenance for Ramsay. Dick had been very unreliable with maintenance right from the start, paying meagre amounts when he felt like it. In the final divorce settlement, Dick was also ordered to pay back R50 000 that he had borrowed from me for a business venture and this he had never done. Now I tried again to get this money out of him. I took him to Maintenance Court and he was ordered to pay but he never did and short of putting him in jail, I could do nothing. I became angry and frustrated.

Bill is a man of peace and generous in the extreme and he urged me to let it go.
"Leave it." He said. "It is really not worth it. Money is worth nothing compared to your peace of mind. Just trust God to work it out."

It was a struggle for me as I tried to let it go but God took the matter in hand in a most remarkable way. We were attending The Bay Community Church here in Muizenberg and our pastor, Jeff Kidwell, had invited Kerry Southey to speak at one of services. She was a lovely lady and much used by God in prophecy and prayer for people.

This particular Sunday she stood up and said the Lord had given her a word for a lady who had been married four times. Now this does not happen very often in Christian circles and I knew immediately it was for me and my spirit receptors quickened.
However then she said, "This lady must forgive her ex husband."
I knew that wasn't me, as God had walked me through that long process of forgiveness but Kerry went on, "No, God

says she has forgiven him, but that she has not told her ex that she has forgiven, and she must do this to release him completely."

Well, I knew that was true so this word was meant for me. God showed me my heart and I had to tell Dick I forgave him and release him from all the money he owed me. I wrote him a letter and sent it with Ramsay who was going to spend the day with his father that day. When Dick received that letter he phoned, weeping as he thanked me. All animosity and anger was dissolved and I was truly free from the bonds of the relationship.

Money is less important than a free heart.

There have still been times here in Cape Town when my tension levels have been too high and I have found myself outside my Airplane and with slight MS symptoms but I have never been admitted to hospital again with any MS-related problems. I just climb back into my Airplane and rest in Him till the symptoms have gone.

When Dick committed suicide last year it was a terrible shock and my heart ached for him. If only he had turned to the Lord in his troubles and not taken his own life.

Stress is a major factor in MS, as I have discovered, and with this trauma I really had to climb into my Airplane and rest in God as the stress was too great. I got symptoms and I did not feel at all well. However the Lord was there in all the sadness of tragedy. Ramsay and his wife, Elena, flew out from Dubai for the funeral and we were able to pick up on the good relationships we had had with Dick's family. We have to trust God in all things even the sorrow of suicide.

Joy and laughter are healing and I am so blessed with Bill who makes me laugh at everything. Now that we are getting older we forget things but just laugh at ourselves. It is so pointless to get upset and angry about little things. A purple ribbon is the sign of support for Alzheimer's and when we have a particularly forgetful moment we say we are wearing our purple ribbons!

We do not have much money and my wonderful children are helping and supporting us and my dear Laurine helps us with my dad's pension. We have learned to trust God for all our needs. Why worry? Worry doesn't help at all and interferes with the joy of relying on God.

God is wonderful and He does perform wonders for the children He loves. He loves us and cares for us in every tiny circumstance. I have proved it.

I am now free and healed. I went back to Groote Schuur Hospital for a check up at the neurology department last year and the doctor said I did not have MS. It must have been an incorrect diagnosis, he said.

I told him about the MRI scan from the Johannesburg General Hospital, which had shown lots of little scabs on my brain. He looked at me doubtfully and said I was now normal and fit. I told him how God had healed me but he obviously thought I was brain damaged in another dimension.

I did not have another MRI scan and I don't know if the scabs are still there but my brain underneath them is healed anyway. That I know. I was diagnosed 40 years ago and it has taken all those years of God working patiently and faithfully, in and with me, to heal me from Multiple Sclerosis.

I am now retired and as fit as a fiddle. I go to exercise classes twice a week and am involved, with my husband, in helping a community nursery school and helping to distribute food to the needy on behalf of our church. In my spare time I love to paint, transferring the beauty of God's creation onto canvas for others to enjoy.

God has not finished with me yet and I hope He still has more for me to do for Him.

Psalm 9:1-2

> I will praise you, Lord, with all my heart,
> I will tell all the wonderful things you have done.
> I will sing for joy because of you.
> I will sing praise to you, Most High.

I thank and praise God for my healing and all the miracles in my life.

LaVergne, TN USA
30 September 2009
159500LV00001B/33/P